OXFORD MEDICAL PUBLICATIONS

**Management in
general practice**

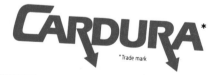

OXFORD GENERAL PRACTICE SERIES

Editorial board

Management in general practice

Oxford General Practice Series 8

PETER PRITCHARD
General practitioner

KENNETH LOW
Management consultant

MERRILL WHALEN
Practice manager

OXFORD   NEW YORK   TORONTO   MELBOURNE

OXFORD UNIVERSITY PRESS

Oxford University Press, Walton Street, Oxford OX2 6DP
Oxford New York Toronto
Delhi Bombay Calcutta Madras Karachi
Petaling Jaya Singapore Hong Kong Tokyo
Nairobi Dar es Salaam Cape Town
Melbourne Auckland

and associated companies in
Berlin Ibadan

Oxford is a trade mark of Oxford University Press

First published 1984
Reprinted 1985, 1986
Reprinted 1987, 1989 (with corrections and update), 1990

British Library Cataloguing in Publication Data

Pritchard, Peter
Management in general practice.—(Oxford general practice series; 8)
1. Medical offices—Great Britain—Management
2. Family medicine—Great Britain
I. Title   II. Low, Kenneth   III. Whalen, Merrill
362.1' 72' 068   R728
ISBN 0-19-261391-X

Library of Congress Cataloging in Publication Data

Pritchard, P. M. M. (Peter M. M.)
Management in general practice.
(Oxford general practice series; no. 8)
Bibliography: p.
Includes index.
1. Family medicine—Practice.   I. Low, Kenneth.
II. Whalen, Merrill.   III. Title.   IV. Series.
R729.5.G4P739   1984   610'.68   83-25164
ISBN 0-19-261391-X (pbk.)

Printed in Great Britain by
St. Edmundsbury Press, Suffolk.

Foreword

By Sir George Godber, GCB, DM, FRCP, FRCGP
Formerly Chief Medical Officer, Department of Health and Social Security

General medical practice was once an uncomplicated one-to-one relationship between a physician and a patient, who sought his help for the treatment of illness or injury; it is so no longer. Medicine in those days was largely empirical and, in honesty, not very effective. In the last half-century the technical content of medicine has greatly increased, diagnosis has become more accurate, and therapy more effective. These factors alone require organization within medical practice.

Paradoxically, the non-medical and even the non-technical components of health care have become more important, and make the better organization of all forms of medical practice imperative. As the introduction says 'teamwork does not just happen when professionals are mixed together'; so it follows that each group needs to analyse how and why teamwork does or does not happen.

General medical practice is the more important because so much health care is highly specialized and requires hospital-based teams. But both the technical and the social components of primary health care have led, inevitably, to a more complex organization of practice. More than four-fifths of general practitioners now work in groups, sharing premises and staff. and working with other professionals, mainly nurses, and with the social services. Team working may vary widely in its pattern, but there is no doubt that it needs organizing. Doctors now have a far more complex and changing body of medical knowledge, with which they must be familiar, and they now use more sophisticated equipment.

A few doctors enjoy administration and do their own, at the expense of the time which they have for practising medicine. All make use of some supporting staff, and all must work with other professions. Many groups now employ an administrator or manager, who needs preparation for the role, and will be better for a wider understanding of primary health care and its relation to the whole NHS, than is likely to be gained from simple on-the-job learning.

This book is, at the same time, a compendium for the established manager or administrator in general practice, and a textbook for trainees. It is not written from the narrow viewpoint of the doctor alone, but attempts to present the needs of the whole primary care team for administrative support. There is much for health professionals to read, even though one of the authors has already written an admirable manual for medical trainees. The range of topics is wide – from fire precautions to the rapidly changing use of computers, as well as problems of team development. Support for the recent development of patient participation is as welcome as it is to be expected in anything with which Peter Pritchard is concerned. Like the Community Health Councils, these groups simply have to be made to work if health care is to be fully acceptable to the public in the future.

This book undoubtedly fills an important gap in the literature of primary health care. It should be of great help, not only to those working in primary care, but also to the planners and managers of the National Health Service. The future of the NHS in Britain depends on getting the best out of each Health District for its own population, despite limited resources. Better-managed primary health care will be the most important factor in that progress. The authors deserve congratulations for the way in which they have undertaken this difficult task.

Preface

To help people to achieve good health is one of the aims of general practice. Ill-health is determined by so many factors – social, psychological, and environ-mental – apart from the disease itself, that the means of achievement of good health go far beyond the traditional boundaries of general practice.

Of necessity, professionals other than doctors must be involved – health visitors, district nurses, social workers, and many others. Teamwork and communication become essential ingredients.

But health is primarily of concern to the individual in his home or work setting, in partnership with the caring professions and their helpers. The choice between health and ill-health may be determined by individual lifestyle and appreciation of risks. Professionals need to understand the subtle equilibria underlying individual choice if they are to influence people to be healthy and to gain full benefit from health services. These complex equilibria determining health are mirrored by the complexity of the interactions within the health-care team, and in its relationship with patients and the world outside. A manager must have a clear understanding of the intricate background to her work.

The primary health-care team, of which the general practitioner (GP) is a key member, is central to this wider concept of health and health care. *Primary health care* is an appropriate title for this activity, which includes promoting health, preventing ill-health, and providing accessible, acceptable, and afford-able health care and rehabilitation, with the full participation of the community. Such a description accords with the World Health Organization (WHO) phil-osophy for modern health care in industrialized countries (Kaprio 1979). Much of this wider view of general practice has already become part of the policy of the Royal College of General Practitioners, with its emphasis on prevention, a sensitive consulting style, and performance review including community participation.

To achieve the WHO goals for primary health care, encompassing general practice, presents a considerable challenge to those involved in managing the service – general practitioners, nurses, practice managers, administrators, receptionists, and so on.

In this book an attempt is made to describe some of the management issues which arise in this complex field. All staff in the practice, and many outside will be involved in this process. General practitioners have a specific management role, but the key person in the day-to-day management of the practice is now the practice manager. This applies particularly to larger practices.

So what is management? Is it an esoteric science shrouded in jargon which no ordinary person can understand? Not in this book, where jargon has been kept to a minimum. Management, in the eyes of the authors, is the *systematic application of common sense and specialized knowledge and skills in order to achieve aims, now and in the future.* The authors attempt to draw on their different knowledge and experience, so the style may vary for different facets of the subject.

GPs talk about clinical management of patients or disease, as well as management of the practice. This text is primarily concerned with practice management, though the two are really interdependent, and the same principles and methods apply to both.

In general practice, the tempo of the work is unique. The tension generated by the urgency of many decisions, and the uncertainty in which the work takes place, require a high standard of management skill in order to keep services running. The achievement of longer term objectives, such as planning or preventive programmes requires an even higher order of ability – to allot priorities and not be too distracted by crises. One hopes that good planning and management will forestall some crises.

Practice managers have a central role – between patients, doctors, nurses, other staff, and the wider environment. They describe themselves as a 'go-between', a 'pig-in-the-middle', and other titles which emphasize that the major part of their role is dealing with people. Hence the first section of seven chapters of the book reflect this concern.

1. In the first chapter a practice manager describes a typical day in her life, from which conclusions are drawn about the dual nature of her job – reacting to other people and situations, while keeping a measure of control, so that objectives are achieved and performance reviewed. Her important role is considered in some detail, as it has not, so far, received the attention it deserves.

2. The practice manager may be responsible for many staff, so she will need technical knowledge, as well as managerial and social skills which are described and discussed in Chapter 2. Relatively new employment legislation has high-lighted the need for the manager to know about it.

3. Communication, as a word, is over-used, describing as it does, the private conversations of two individuals, or doctor and patient, or addressing a group, or writing to consultants. In a large practice, the sense of identity may be lost if communication is poor. If messages are not passed on, then lives are put at risk. Some ways of communicating and facilitating are described in Chapter 3. A discussion of group interactions is included, to help the practice manager to observe and influence the processes of the group of which she is a member.

4. An essential part of managing is learning and teaching. The practice manager will have to teach her own staff, and may have to arrange suitable training courses for them. She will also need to give management support to a trainee general practitioner, who must be given an opportunity to learn about management in practice. These topics are considered in Chapter 4.

5. Team-working does not just happen when professionals are mixed together. In Chapter 5 the nature of team-working is explored, and ways of learning about it, and improving team effectiveness are discussed.

6. Patients crop up in every chapter, but in Chapter 6 mutual attitudes are explored. Patients' needs and rights to information are discussed, and ways of co-operating, for example patient participation groups, are described.

7. The practice manager will probably be able to take much of the load of management off the shoulders of the doctor, who can then get on with the work only he (or she) can do. But there are certain mangement functions in which the doctor has an essential part to play, such as determining policies, planning, and decision-making. The practice manager's and the doctor's roles are different, but complementary. These issues are taken up in Chapter 7.

8. The second section of the book is about services and systems, but we still cannot deal with them in isolation from the people involved. Chapter 8 is about the reception of patients, and the problems which may arise. Accessibility is the key factor in any service to the public, add the factor of urgency, and the need for acceptability, and the result is a very complex interaction in which management skills are essential. The receptionist's role and the skills she needs are also explored.

9. Prescribing is a controversial and important part of general practice: it is also costly, and is an area of high risk. Ways in which the practice manager can help are discussed – particularly in arranging that information is available, and that fail-safe systems are devised – for example for repeat prescriptions. The management of dispensing is omitted for lack of space.

10. With an ageing population, and other factors which increase the demand for a doctor's services, the need for prevention becomes more urgent. This approach should also improve people's health and the quality of their lives. It is easy to make statements like this, but to turn them into practical action is complex and difficult. Ways of achieving a higher level of prevention are explored in Chapter 10, and in the first four appendices.

11. Medical records fulfil a variety of functions which are outlined in Chapter 11. The development of a practical record system is discussed. All those working in a practice, as well as patients, need access to information specific for their needs – often at short notice. Ways of meeting these needs with modern information systems and libraries are discussed. The services of a librarian may be the key which unlocks this information.

12. Computers are a powerful tool in the handling of information. Their advantages and limitations are discussed, particularly in the context of the practice manager's role. Computers will not make bad records good, so essential steps before computerization are considered in detail.

13. A general practice functions as a business, and must make a profit if it is to survive. Efficiency is essential, so that money is not wasted; but more important is the balance between money spent and value received in terms of services to patients, or patients' health. Can this 'cost-effectiveness' equation be solved?

14. The third section of the book considers objects – first the building. For those content with their premises, there are problems with maintenance, security, administration, and finance. For those who want to move or improve their premises, there are formidable tasks in relation to design, finance, and moving. Chapter 14 gives an account of these topics, and references where further information may be sought.

15. Equipment to support practice management may be highly complex, and exploit the advances in microprocessors. This topic is discussed in Chapter 15.

16. In the final section of this book an attempt is made to apply existing knowledge of organization and management to general practice. The characteristics of different organizational structures and the problems they are likely to generate are considered in Chapter 16, along with an approach to problem solving.

17. Planning is a constant theme of the book, and this is dealt with in more detail in Chapter 17. Models and check-lists for planning are considered. Planning takes place at a number of levels from the practice to the national or international level. For resources to be used effectively, these plans must be integrated if possible. The GP may have a part to play at all levels.

18. The main aim of this book might be seen as encouraging people to look at the way they do things – to consider whether their present approach is the best, to review performance, and seek improvements, and to be sensitive to other people's feelings, and to changes both inside the organization and in the outside world. Review of performance at individual and group level, and what is needed in tems of attitudes, and methods is considered in the final chapter.

Appendices. A book of this size can give only a small fraction of the information needed for managing a practice. The emphasis has been more on ways of finding out. In addition to the four appendices of procedures for prevention, there are three which contain information for patients, useful addresses, and a list for further reading on management. Many references appear in the text for easier access, as well as at the end of the book.

Apology. Not all practice managers are female, and not all doctors and patients are male, and it is only for ease of reading that the feminine gender is used for the first and the masculine for the others. The authors hope that this economical device will not cause offence.

Oxford   P. P.
November 1983   K. L.
                                                                                                              M. W.

Acknowledgements

We are grateful to many people who have contributed information and ideas.

In particular we should like to thank Shirely Elliott, Bill Fraser, Ekke Kuenssberg, Joan Mant, and Wendy Pritchard for commenting on the typescript; and Lex Barr, Norman Ellis, Elaine Fullard, Janet Hobbs, Tony Leahy, Beryl Martin, Donald Mungall, Jane Norman, and June Raine who have contributed useful ideas and comments.

We are indebted to the practitioners at West Granton Medical Group for their generosity in giving one of us (M.W.) the time to write.

Several librarians have assisted us, in particular Enid Leonard, Angela Hornby, and Joan Hammond. Pamela Beardsley typed the manuscript.

We are grateful to Sir George Godber for the stimulus his work has given to us, and for writing the Foreword.

Contents

SECTION B **SERVICES AND SYSTEMS**

SECTION C **'THINGS'**

SECTION D **APPLICATION OF MANAGEMENT THEORY**

Abbreviations

BMA	British Medical Association
BNF	British National Formulary
CAB	Citizens' Advice Bureau
CHC	Community Health Council
CSM	Committee on Safety of Medicines
DGM	District General Manager
DHA	District Health Authority
DHSS	Department of Health and Social Security†
DMO	District Medical Officer (formerly District Community Physician)
FPC	Family Practitioner Committee
GP	General Medical Practitioner
GPFC	General Practice Finance Corporation
HV	Health Visitor
LMC	Local Medical Committee
MIMS	*Monthly Index of Medical Specialities*
NHS	National Health Service
PHC	Primary Health Care
RCGP	Royal College of General Practitioners
RCN	Royal College of Nurses
RHA	Regional Health Authority
SFA	*Statement of fees and allowances* (The 'Red Book')
WHO	World Health Organization

†Now Department of Health (1988)

Section A

People and management

1 The practice manager

Tucked away in a desk drawer, the practice manager's job description may serve as a useful guide should the extent of her authority or responsibility ever be in question. What it will not convey is the shifting pattern of daily events which characterizes any general practice trying to provide a round-the-clock service for patients.

The aim of this chapter is to enable the reader to identify the basic features of the role as represented by the 'day in the life of a practice manager'. Comment and analysis follow to help the reader judge how closely this particular model fits reality, whilst recognizing that no ideal exists. Variations on the theme will, of course, apply according to circumstances, such as the number of partners; whether the practice is rural, urban, or inner-city; the numbers and kinds of patients; the building itself and its accessibility, and so on.

In taking a look at a practice manager in action we hope to create for the reader a sense of what is possible as well as desirable in the management of primary care.

A DAY IN THE LIFE OF A PRACTICE MANAGER

It's raining again, with a driving cold east wind. 'If you can live in these parts you can live anywhere'. I am not certain of the quotation's origins, but whoever said it is perfectly correct! The car radio tells me 'it is 8.25 precisely'. I think I will stop off *en route* and buy the morning paper. It is ridiculous to read the newspaper at 11 o'clock in the evening. After all, I could read the paper with my morning coffee. I smile to myself at how far apart theory and practice are, no matter how hard we try, but I don't stop and drive straight to the surgery.

I lock up the car and run head down to take quick shelter in reception but not before the almond tree showers me and I am soaked. I must make a point of seeing our gardener this week and ask him to cut off these lower branches.

Betty's smile always greets me and warms me first thing in the morning. (I must remember when talking to trainee general practitioners next week on the subject of selecting staff to mention 'smile'.)

8.50 a.m. Betty, our full-time receptionist and I have a talk about what today holds in store for us.

1. Availability of appointments. (I know that Betty has made a decision, and quite correctly so, to request some extra consulting time from Dr Jones in the afternoon, particularly so as she points out that Monday's appointment sheets are becoming heavily booked already.) Dr Jones has telephoned to say that he is visiting a patient who is terminally ill and hopes to be at the surgery by 10 a.m. Betty is to mention to the doctor when he arrives that she is requesting a few extra appointments, preferably at the end of his scheduled Friday afternoon consulting time.

2. Availability of doctors. Dr Brown is attending a meeting in the afternoon, which commences at 2.30 p.m. He will therefore, not be able to undertake home visit requests in the afternoon. I note with reassurance Betty's neat handwriting on the top right-hand section of the Visits Book 'Dr Brown unavailable all afternoon'.

3. Medical Secretary student. I am informed that Miss Clarke, a second year student in medical secretarial studies, who is undertaking her field work at the practice, is polite at all times, does know the alphabet and can therefore file, is interested in learning, and is a most keen student. We agree that Miss Clarke may answer the appointments telephone in reception for the remainder of the morning, under Betty's most excellent supervision. In the afternoon it is hoped that the student will take out the appropriate medical records for surgery, thereafter if time permits, have a 'teach-in' session with Grace, part-time receptionist of long-standing who has agreed to spend time with Miss Clarke to explain patient registrations, completion of the multitude of forms, and the age–sex register. 'Not too much too quickly, remember', but I stop myself there as even I think I am sounding like an old mother hen.

I suggest that Miss Clarke and I have coffee together on Tuesday of next week. I would like to listen to her talking: her observations – and I hope she will feel free to criticize. I inform her that a 'newcomers' views can prove quite enlightening and invaluable. I think I reassure her.

4. Meeting with architect and 'telephone man' in the staff-room at 2.30 p.m. Betty nods approvingly when I mention the meeting and directs her eyes to the calendar. I often wonder who is briefing whom in these morning sessions. I am happy with the relationship and know that it is with mutual respect that we cover the days 'predictable' happenings by talking them over in this way.

We both know that our morning *tête-à-tête* is complete. I collect the mail and she turns her attention to her student. 'We have ten patients called James Wilson, some of them father and son, so you must carefully check name, address, date of birth . . .'

9.00 a.m. I feel a little uneasy. The telephone is making a noise of sorts, but more of a 'ping' than its correct ring. I think that reception is trying to put through a telephone call on my extension. All is quiet . . . I open the mail. I begin to look at the headlines on the front page of a medical journal and am about to turn to page 47 to follow the story but stop myself and continue opening the mail. We practice managers all feel guilty about 'reading' at work – why? I read the mail and place it on clips: immediate action, pending, for reading at home, accounts, etc. The quarterly statement from the Family Practitioner Committee (FPC)† I place on 'pending' but then decide it is sensible to take action immediately and enter it in my statistics book. It takes approximately ten minutes and I am also interested in making a quick observation to compare the figures with those of the previous quarter. I note that Dr Fraser's list in the 'over 75 year old' category has risen dramatically, which I would imagine is a reflection on the fact that many of the houses in the practice area have been recently modernized and adapted as 'sheltered housing' for the elderly and infirm. I am delighted to note that the vaccination and immunization figures continue to rise. The night-visit item has shown a considerable reduction? I would like to spend a great deal longer on this, but meantime I am dealing with the mail. I remind myself that I must get down to compiling full practice statistics – consultations, home visits, overnight calls, weekend work, baby clinics, antenatal clinics . . . and I think of the crucial importance of this information and the many hours of necessary discussion, deliberations, and action that will follow when in a position to sit around a table and look at the evidence of this practice's workload and of course service to the patients.

---

† In Scotland the functions of the FPC are undertaken by Health Boards, and in Northern Ireland by Health and Social Services Boards.

'Ping' . . . this most definitely is not the normal noise the telephone makes. The receptionist meets me *en route*. The heavy rain gets the blame – we have had trouble before. Apparently only an occasional call is coming through.

'Engineer, this is a doctors' surgery. May we have priority given to our telephone fault' . . . I suggest that the receptionist informs me in approximately 15 minutes if full telephone facility is not restored.

10.00 a.m. I have asked a typewriter salesman to call. I do not wish to waste his time, nor mine. I know the model that I think I would like to purchase. It has been well tested and our typists report back favourably. 'Mr Rollinson, good morning to you. We like your company's machine very much but I would like information on the following':

(1) the cost of purchasing – including VAT;
(2) the cost of leasing – over three years, five years, or eight years;
(3) maintenance costs (would the firm consider maintenance under a group price for all typewriters within the practice?);
(4) details of after-sales service (and I stress with him the importance of this issue. Would he be able to ensure a temporary replacement typewriter if the original had to be returned to the workshop for repair, for example?);
(5) what discount, if any;
(6) part exchange.

I make the coffee whilst he gets his papers together. He is ready with the answers and I take notes. As a good salesman, Mr Rollinson suggests I type out the order now, but I decide to wait and think it over. He is amiable and departs saying that he will be hearing from me. No doubt he will. I am satisfied that it was the correct thing to do to invite the salesman to call, rather than discuss all the various options over the telephone. A typewriter at some £700 is a major item of equipment and I have a page full of notes on information which will need digesting and discussing with the partners. I may telephone the accountant to ask his advice about leasing equipment. That awful word 'cash flow', but I ponder for a moment trying to weigh up outright purchase against leasing.

10.30 a.m. I remember reading an article on coping with stress or some such title where it suggested writing a work-list prior to leaving the office each evening, listing all the issues you want reminding of – anything in fact that is on your mind. The article gave examples for the working wife. It may be to remember to buy a loaf of bread, or to draft the minutes of the finance meeting. I had laughed at the time but it could have been my list. Simplicity itself, but for me it works! It heads my action tray and today reads numbers 1–27 and that's average. One is Mrs Blair's salary. Mrs Blair, our cleaning lady, is into her fifth week off sick. Her contract, as for any other member of staff, states that in the event of sickness and absence from work, full salary will be paid for a period of four weeks, thereafter at the discretion of the doctors. I meet the doctors today at our weekly working lunch and I will mention this. Checking the records I note that Mrs Blair has been with the practice for over seven years and has had excellent attendance. I am confident that I will be able to inform her that the doctors will continue to pay her wages in the meantime, and a note in the diary reminds me to visit Mrs Blair next week.

10.40 a.m. Item number two is staff holidays. On top of the action file is a sheaf of requests from the staff regarding holidays. How can we think about spring holidays when winter is still with us. I can dismiss this instantly since the staff have dutifully written down their holiday dates, allowing me plenty of time to draw up relief and extra duty rotas. It takes fully half an hour to put up the various colour bars indicating absences from the practice, on the wall-hung holiday planner and to work out a suggested rota for extra duty and holiday cover.

I suppose it took months, perhaps even longer, to persuade everyone that I am only too delighted to discuss anything with them face to face, and of course I would prefer it that way, but please, please everyone, can you write down issues such as holiday dates so that I have something in front of me to work from, and not to have to depend entirely on memory.

Next for action: a written request from the health visitors and nursing sisters for a lunch-time meeting with doctors, primarily to discuss the outcome of the influenza protection programme for elderly patients and those at risk. Facts and figures were taken throughout the late autumn/winter period to enable assessment to take place, with a view to improving the service offered at the onset of next winter. I suggest a likely date, enter it in the diary, type out a memo with the details of day, time, place of meeting, and decide to meet the health visitors and nurses to give them their copy. We all agree that a fair degree of preparation is required before the meeting and I don't need reminding of the disastrous occasion when last we met formally, totally unprepared. I reassure myself that I won't let it happen again! I suggest that if the health visitors and nurses would be kind enough to note down information, statistics, etc., I will be only too happy to have these typed and photocopied for circulation, prior to the meeting. Back at the office I remember to telephone the lady who will prepare a light lunch on the day of the meeting, and a note to remind myself to pay for the lunches.

11.30 a.m. The secretary knocks – 'May I do some photocopying'. She is tense, pale, and tired looking. I have noticed it before, but decide to remain silent unless approached.

Then the new GP trainee comes in. Dr Forbes has been with the practice one week now. She asks me about courses she wishes to attend, what Section 63 means, her removal expenses, and whether she can have a telephone extension for her bedroom now that she is soon to go on duty overnight.

The telephone rings. It is Dr Wood: 'My home visits are unusually light this morning and I would like to discuss a suggestion for changes in my consulting time-table. Will you be there in about half an hour?' I tell him that around 12.00 will be suitable and I am just on the point of putting the receiver down when I hear him say hurriedly 'and I have a change of dates for my holidays also. Please remind me to give you the new dates'.

As to the trainee's request, I know it will be far quicker to deal with them all myself and present her with a *fait accompli,* but I know that it would be quite wrong not to spend some time right now relieving her anxiety. We spend more than 30 minutes together filling in forms to apply for courses, speaking to the finance officer at the Family Practitioner Committee with regard to removal expenses, and setting the wheels in motion for provision of a telephone extension by telephoning the appropriate department. I go over the 'Red Book' (Statement of Fees and Allowances) pointing out the relevant paragraphs. The trainee tells me that she feels very uneasy about the prospect of managing a practice when the time comes. We agree to meet and spend a full afternoon together discussing practice organization and management. I point out a course that I noted in a journal that would appear to be very relevant and photocopy the details for her. The telephone rings but just before answering and as the trainee departs, I give her a copy of a typed list of all members of staff, their respective hours of duty and roles, the names of the health visitors, and the nursing sisters attached to the practice. 'Another week and you will begin to know who's who' – I try to sound reassuring.

I answer the telephone call and speak to a medical officer from the Department of Health. He asks me to discuss with the doctors the possibility of a group of doctors and nurses from overseas visiting the practice. To fit in with their very tight schedule it will have to be Wednesday afternoon. The group would like an opportunity to visit a general practice and hear at grass root level about primary medical care in this country and speak to the general practitioners, health visitors, and nursing sisters. As it happens Wednesday would in fact be appropriate – 4.00 p.m. following the well baby clinic when all will be present, but I will confirm arrangements by telephoning back in the late afternoon.

Dr Wood arrives and apologises for being late – I had not noticed. He puts his suggestion to me about changes in consultation times. We look at the *whole* position, the workload for the receptionists, the availability of consulting rooms, and not the doctors' position in isolation. We see that we can slightly rearrange the consulting timetable and this is now most acceptable to the patients, the receptionists, to the doctor, and to his colleagues. Looking at the doctors' holiday planner we discover that his proposal to change holiday dates will cause endless difficulties. Dr Wood agrees that we have a problem. I'm genuinely sympathetic and, I am certain that if we discuss it with his colleagues it will work out satisfactorily for all in the end.

12.30 p.m. I write down the items that require discussion with the partners over lunch.

12.45 p.m. The second delivery of mail has arrived. The proof of our new letter-heads has been sent for checking. I note an important mistake in a telephone number. Clearly marking the error I am about to send it back to the printers when I remember that we had endless problems some three years back, when our 'How to See Your Doctor' cards were printed with one particular line stating 'a.m.' instead of 'p.m.' I ask the secretary to read this over carefully and I will collect it after lunch. Two heads are better than one on such occasions!

1.00 p.m. Barely an hour to go over all the various issues that I would like to discuss with the doctors and only Dr Wood and myself have arrived. I'm mildly irritated but inwardly understand what it must be like to have a fully booked surgery plus 'extra patients' (including a tragic case of four little ones who must be examined before going into care), and a larger than normal home visits list, not to mention trying hard to arrive back at the surgery to meet your partners by 1.00 p.m.

Dr Wood asks about the progress I am making with an organized in-service training programme for staff. Members of staff all agreed that they would like to attend a series of evening sessions and I have worked out a draft programme. 'Are we beginning next week then?' he aks enthusiastically. 'Doctor, I need time to write to invited speakers, arrange loan of video and slide projector, encourage our health visitors and sisters to give a talk on the role that they undertake in the primary care team – and lots more!' 'Never thought of that side of it – but do you know, it's a jolly good idea. It will work like clockwork when our staff are trained into our ways!' (I think just wait until a good discussion group gets into full flight at one of these proposed meetings and we'll see that the training and benefit is not one sided! – assuming of course that I can persuade the doctors that they too must assist by being present and participating in group work and discussion.)

1.25 p.m. All the doctors of the group have arrived. I have eaten, therefore I ask if I may discuss one or two points with them:

1. Decision on the typewriter. I present the full details.
2. Mrs Blair's salary while off sick.
3. The proposed changes in Dr Wood's consulting timetable.
4. Arrangements for the forthcoming Monday holiday – medical and staffing arrangements. Rather stupid of me but I have forgotten to have with me the figures and information on the corresponding Monday holiday of last year. Dr George remembers, however, and we are left in no doubt that it was almost impossible for one partner to 'cope'. We agree to have a clear notice placed in the waiting room indicating the arrangements for the Monday holiday and for the notice to be placed today.
5. Visitors from abroad.
6. Doctors/health visitors/nursing sisters' working lunch-time meeting on 'influenza'.

7. Sister will be going on a middle management course and her relief will commence on . . . (Dr Cranley mumbles that he has never heard of such nonsense as a management course for nurses. His colleagues tease him good humouredly.)

We are about to disperse at 2.10 p.m. (rather late actually and I am glad that Grace telephoned the staff-room to let us know that three patients are now waiting for Dr Jones – and is Dr Brown remembering that she has to be in town for a meeting at 2.30 p.m.?). Dr Gray asks if I have a minute to talk. One of his patients had complained to him about the appointments receptionist's attitude and apparent disregard for his request for an urgent appointment. The full facts must be sought and I can make no comment until I hear the complete story.

2.20 p.m. It will be ten minutes before the meeting will start so I decide to wait in reception. It gives me the opportunity to make enquiries about the patient's complaint. The receptionist who had been involved is now off duty and this important and worrying issue will, therefore, have to wait until Monday morning.

Grace approaches with a broad smile and a large envelope in her hands, 'The wedding photographs!' and for a few minutes we put all thoughts of work away and hand round the photographs of her son's wedding. We talk for a moment or two about our children and I am prompted to ask Betty about her daughter who has just begun her nurse training at the local general hospital. Anne, the secretary, has been polite in joining in the conversation but is definitely preoccupied and quick to return to her typewriter. I overhear Anne mutter to herself that she will be thankful to complete Dr Fraser's tape. 'I think he must dictate in the car because there is a tremendous amount of background noise, like traffic, and it is almost impossible for me to hear properly!' Talking of audio equipment has reminded me that an invitation was sent to the practice to attend an exhibition of office equipment to be held in a hotel in town on Wednesday of next week and I am certain that Anne and I could attend and then have lunch together. She appears to be enthusiastic. 'Agreed then.' (Something *is* worrying Anne and making her irritable.)

2.30 p.m. The architect and the telephone man arrive and as they do the receptionist passes on a call from Dr Wood, the partner who has a particular interest in the new surgery extension and who is to join the meeting. He has been called out to visit a patient urgently and asks me to start. I am looking forward to the meeting. Plans and sketches and a computerized telephone system are a new world to me and it is exciting. The partners agreed to go ahead with the surgery extension financed through the General Practice Finance Corporation, under the cost rent, and improvement grant schemes. The design in general is approved and we must now look seriously at our requirements for telephone equipment. For almost half an hour I am bombarded with questions. I can answer some, but the vast majority I cannot. It soon becomes apparent that we need to undertake a fairly extensive study of the telephone load. Our present equipment will most definitely need to be extended, if not renewed. Dr Wood joins us and we brief him. We listen, and I am trying extremely hard to understand the telephone man, but he is far too technical. We ask him to explain in plain language the modern 'desk top' type of equipment. It is almost 4.00 p.m. and we go over what action each of us must take in order to be fully prepared for our next meeting. We have talked through the problem, but in fact wasted some time since I was not fully prepared for this meeting. I have taken notes and am planning already how to set about a study of the telephone load.

4.05 p.m. A blissful cup of tea. The telephone rings: the receptionist at the branch surgery reports a 'choked' drain outside the building but well within the surgery boundary. Where will I find a plumber at 4.00 p.m. on a Friday afternoon? What would I do without my 'friends of the practice list' (plumber, joiner, electrician)? Eddie groans a little when I call him but agrees to leave immediately. I take the opportunity of asking if he would mind having a look at the drains of both premises – not today to course, I add cheekily.

4.20 p.m. I had hoped to get a newsletter for the practice out today. I decide to list all the items to be included. I remember that only last week I received a delightful letter from an elderly housebound patient wishing to thank the reception staff for all their help and a special thank you to the lady who takes her repeat prescription request. I retrieve the letter from the filing basket and read from it 'her caring, understanding voice always makes me feel much better . . .' I decide to conclude the newsletter with the old lady's letter. It speaks for itself.

The telephone rings; and as it does I am reminded that I promised to be in touch this afternoon with the doctor who requested the visit of overseas doctors and nurses. It is indeed he, and we finalize the details for the visit.

It is almost 5.00 p.m. I am tempted to take the next item off the action file. I do, but only to flick over the papers. I am reassured that while there are definitely pressing issues, Monday for some, and the next day for others will do. I check the diary for Monday.

It is still raining, but this time I avoid the almond tree. The branch surgery is less than a mile distant and I decide to look in on my way home. Everything is running smoothly – apart from Eddie who is muttering under his breath but definitely getting to grips with the problem. 'It's them paper towels going down the loo – can't you tell the doctors it's time they got one of the modern fixed in the wall hand drying machines!'

I am pleased to hear from the receptionist that the new method of recording home visits is proving to be efficient and a great improvement on the 'old' system. I congratulate Nora who had the initiative to suggest this alternative system.

5.40 p.m. I drive home, and as I do, reflect on the day. Perhaps I would award myself a 7 out of 10 day today. I could do better – and will, perhaps on Monday.

Electrically operated hand driers? The patient who had made a complaint? We'll need someone to monitor the telephone load for a week? In-service training programme? The secretary . . . I do hope she is not wanting to leave us?

Comments on the practice manager's day

If we now look at our practice manager's busy Friday perhaps the most significant feature was the degree to which she was able to retain control despite the various demands upon her time. She did more than cope because she was able to *manage* the day's events instead of allowing them to control her. She was not simply reacting to whatever pressure was next brought to bear. She was able to initiate action herself. How did she do this?

Reaction and action

She had a full and complicated day but we can pick out some elements which provided a structure to the day and which helped her to remain in control. Even the early and apparently trivial incident with the dripping almond tree provides an example of how a manager can be on the lookout for opportunities to take initiatives. Instead of waiting for complaints she decided to act herself, in this case through delegating a simple job. Not a bad sequence for a manager to take as a model – first the reaction, then a decision to have something done; the allocation of responsibility (clear and firm, too, in this instance!); and after the action a check to make sure that what had been intended was implemented. Let us hope the mental note which was her understandable response to a wet reception was sufficient to ensure action and that neither the practice manager nor her colleagues now receive a shower as they arrive at work.

Planning

Mental notes, however, can frequently prove an inadequate way of dealing with intended action. When our manager had to attend a meeting later that day with the general practitioners she made a note beforehand of the items which had to be discussed. Even such basic and simple aids to management as a note-pad and a diary can assist her to discipline any random thoughts or requests. A daily list of things to be done, which is revised and amended as priorities change, helps her to be systematic and can reduce the sense of pressure upon her time. Like the indispensable wall-chart which was used to record holiday dates, a diary is a good example of a simple but effective planning tool; both enabled her to know at a glance what commitments had been made. There is something quite reassuring about a visible expression of what has been decided. Indeed, if long-term requirements are not formally recorded then short-term dissension, leading to problems, accusations of favouritism even, can be the result. Holidays, to take the specific example, represent individual wishes leading to individual arrangements, once agreement has been reached.

If, to quote one management textbook (Stewart 1979), a manager's responsibility is not only to plan and to organize but also to motivate or encourage people at work, then she cannot afford to discount the plans which staff as private people are entitled to make. Positive feelings towards work are inspired by more than pats on the shoulder. A good manager gains the respect of her staff by taking the trouble to back up agreed plans with efficient systems and procedures which will ensure the implementation of ideas. Our practice manager tried to accommodate the different needs of individuals as her later discussion with the doctor showed, but she would have been unable to do so without this blend of humanity and effective but simple administration. Attitudes to work and to one's colleagues are rooted in down-to-earth, practical considerations as well as in psychology.

The diary

Like all aids to good management the practice manager's diary and her daily list were only useful in so far as they helped her to make choices about what had to be done and in what order. The manager still retained control of the day's events because she could decide whether her diary was to be a rigid time-table of planned activity or whether it allowed her sufficient space to be flexible in order to make changes or additions. Diaries are neutral; people decide. Our manager was not to know in advance, as no day can be totally predictable and especially in general practice, that one of the partners would find himself free of commitments and would want to talk about changing his times of consultation and – almost as an afterthought – his own holiday dates. The manager knew that in any daily routine it is still important to find time to be available to one's colleagues. A diary, therefore, not only records what has been agreed beforehand, it allows one to plan uncommitted time. Free time (so-called) in a manager's day does not just happen: it too is the result of planning. A manager has to be disciplined with herself as well as with others; there is nearly always somebody with good intentions waiting to gobble up the available minutes.

One school of thought holds that we engage in frenzied activity, filling up our diaries for example, and rushing about in a harassed manner, precisely because this is *easier* than actually sitting down to choose how we allocate our energies and to plan accordingly. Of course crises will occur and practice managers like everyone else directly involved, will leap into action. But on occasions one can feel that *crisis management*, as it is called, becomes the only mode of response because that is what we are accustomed to and probably what we do well. Do we sometimes wish a crisis upon ourselves and feel secretly relieved that we can respond urgently to an unexpected happening rather than maintain the discipline of the diary? A daily time-table can be a flexible plan, and in medical practice has to be so; but it is the practice manager who can exert the most significant influence in creating a climate where planning is an accepted norm.

Managing as teaching

Back to our practice manager and the doctor whose focus, no doubt after a morning's sequence of anxious patients, was mainly on his own ideas about the changes he wished to discuss. The manager's role in making herself available was not to accede automatically to what was proposed. It was rather to help the doctor see that his needs would inevitably influence and be influenced by those of colleagues. By being attentive, sympathetic even, she helped the doctor to see his wishes in a different perspective, but was able to do so only because she was also being an efficient manager, using her knowledge of planned arrangements (consultation times, holidays) to complement her undoubted humanity. Practice management must provide 'efficiency with a human face' if it is to respond adequately to the needs of both the patients and the people whose range of skills provides the health-care service.

In one sense the practice manager was not only doing her job according to her job description; she was also taking on a complementary role of an informal teacher – helping others to learn from an experience. She is in a good position, having access to the different groups which comprise the practice, to point out what may be the consequences of their actions. Because she is aware of the many influences upon the practice, she may be the best person to help her colleagues learn what kind of behaviour produces good results and what does not. She knows that dissatisfaction can have its origins in a thoughtless action, and therefore she tries to be alert to whatever might be happening in and around the practice. Our practice manager certainly saw this as very much a part of her management responsibility. She exercised her teaching role not only by making sure, patiently, that others understood what was required, but also through example. The practice manager can be an important model whose own ways of exercising sensitivity in combination with care for administrative detail can be adapted by her colleagues.

Being prepared

Meetings inspire love–hate reactions in most of us. While we recognize that decisions which involve numbers of people may require discussion and consultation, our experience is that we often waste time; that we feel uncomfortable if we are ill-prepared; and that we are bored to tears by the meandering drift of the talk. Sometimes, as with our crisis management reactions, even when no crises exists we make use of meetings as a means to *avoid* a problem or a difficulty. How often do we find it easier to bury the nettle in chatter rather than to grasp it?

But our manager knew what she wanted from her lunchtime meeting. She had done her homework and so was able to help herself and the partners to achieve results. She had prepared an agenda, knew her facts in advance (e.g. about the member of staff who had been absent ill), made notes of what was agreed and who would implement the specific points for action. It was a good example of the value of preparation and how some of the weight can be taken off busy doctors.

The meeting with the telephone engineer was different in purpose and style. The engineer's aim was to reach as rapid a conclusion as possible (one could understand *his* motivation), but the manager's aim was to avoid an inappropriately hasty decision – after all (as with the typewriter), investment in capital equipment was under consideration. Time, while important, was not the dominant factor from the practice viewpoint. Further questions, noted by the manager, were to be examined before agreement could be reached. In this kind of meeting a practice manager can best be prepared, not so much with reams of information, but by knowing what she wanted to achieve and by keeping an open mind throughout the discussion.

Clarity of purpose

Not every meeting has to be cut and dried in order to give a sense of achievement. The manager should be aware of the purpose of each meeting – for example whether to record and agree plans for action or to take soundings and then return after an interval. The value of some meetings lies precisely in the opportunity they afford to explore ideas and feelings, which in turn may lead to the decision that further work needs to be done – the logging of phone calls, for instance, which our practice manager felt she had to implement in order to know the facts. Again, a manager who has responsibility for meetings as a means of communication between interested parties must find the right balance between flexibility which can encourage discussion, and rigidity, which insists on adherence to the agenda no matter what else may have happened since it was prepared. The quality of the decisions made will largely depend on the clarity of purpose which she has in setting up the different meetings.

Despite her sense of disappointment, there was, however, an important difference between her two meetings that Friday. One cannot expect to organize right to the last detail; time and space have also to be allowed – planned that is – for further thoughts and for reviewing events.

Thinking ahead

How far can crises be prevented by time to think ahead? A vital part of any manager's role is to encourage the practice to monitor its progress from time to time in order to be able to project its thoughts and ideas towards future plans.

This can be seen as an integral part of a manager's job – to assist with practice audit. Being prepared implies being knowledgeable about what has happened previously. This not only meant that our practice manager wished that she had a record of one of the previous year's holiday Mondays. She also saw it as her responsibility to have the facts and figures to assess the autumn influenza protection programme for elderly patients and those at risk. Without this kind of information a practice cannot know whether its efforts are achieving results.

Evaluation or feedback is not only a question of following the correct administrative procedures. These are augmented by less formal methods; patients too are a source of information which can be assessed and used by an alert practice manager.

The practice newsletter was used to show the gratitude which an elderly patient felt, and was a way for the manager to let staff see how their efforts were appreciated. The feelings which the patient expressed at having received kind attention were no doubt genuine, but to support the professional medical care there must have been good administrative procedures, without which no practice could run efficiently. A follow-up system to ensure home and hospital visits is a necessary adjunct to any well-intentioned policy to provide care for patients. Efficient administration is essential to the management of health care. This is why a practice needs to be able to evaluate how effective it is in providing a service to its patients, and therefore it relies on the manager to record information which must be readily accessible and up to date. Satisfied patients and well-motivated staff who know their job are the best measures of a well-run practice; one which reviews its progress, learns from its experience, and thinks ahead about possible new or different action.

Nobody is perfect

Why, we may wonder, did our manager award herself only 7 out of 10 at the end of that Friday: what did she feel she had failed to do? Perhaps, after all, the mental note about the almond tree was insufficient and she simply forgot it in the ensuing bustle of activity. The meeting about telephones seemed to niggle her a bit because she thought herself not as well-prepared as she would have wished. Or perhaps she wondered whether she might have asked one of her colleagues to take some of the detailed work off her busy shoulders? But then nobody is perfect, not even a well-organized practice manager. She is, thank goodness, not *only* but *mainly* human. Like her colleagues in the practice she will have been aware, too, during the busy day that other demands were waiting to be made upon her resources.

THE NATURE OF THE ROLE

What lessons can be drawn from the description of a busy day in the life of the practice manager? If this was a not untypical experience are there any general principles which can apply to the role of practice manager? To be sure, no ideal model exists in some mythical practice where there are no crises, where patients are rarely ill, and where well-laid plans are never frustrated. The real world consists of continuously ringing telephones, patients anxiously waiting in reception, doctors hastening to emergencies and – of course – blocked drains on Friday afternoons. A kind of structure does emerge, however, which can help both experienced and aspiring practice managers to progress beyond the mere coping stage towards the possibility of control over events.

The main focus, however the role is perceived, is upon people, whether they be in the treatment room, in the waiting room, or behind the formidable consulting room door. The role of manager implies a concern for all the people involved in health care.

This means that the manager must be in a position to have her finger on the pulse of the practice. She has a central role, and, as we have seen she carries out her responsibilities to people by *planning, organizing, motivating,* and *evaluating.* These are not separate activities but are all of a piece if the practice is to work as an integrated unit. When, for instance, our practice manager agreed to set aside a whole afternoon to discuss practice organization with a trainee, having beforehand prepared a typed list of all staff for the newcomer, she was fulfilling simultaneously the first three functions. Doubtless there followed a subsequent indication by the trainee of how effective she had been, and so the fourth function would also have been met – evaluation. However, we could claim that these functions have general application to management wherever it operates. What are the special features of a practice manager's role which define its particular nature? Firstly, the word 'role' does seem to imply playing a part in a scene written by someone else. Perhaps this is not a bad way to think of what, in effect, a practice manager does, instead of making a sterile list of jobs to be carried out as if they were in isolation from other people's roles. The idea of a role covers not only *what* one has to do but the *way* in which one works. The emphasis is upon sets of relationships between the actors, as it were, on the stage. 'Role description' might be a better way to note what one does day-to-day than job description. Practice managers make a strong point of saying that what is important for them in their work is the making of decisions which impinge upon human beings and which influence relationships. Figure 1.1 shows the manager at the centre of a number of such influences, which include the fabric and the paper-work requirements, as well as people. They each affect in some way how people will respond to one another and to events.

Table 1.1 takes a closer look at the principal elements expressed by the segments of the diagram and how the manager relates, simultaneously and continuously to them.

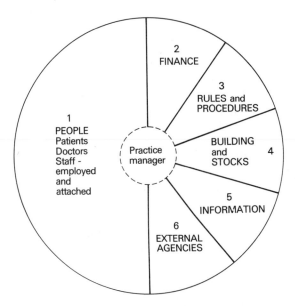

Fig. 1.1. Role of the practice manager.

Knowledge and skills

A number of different kinds of *knowledge* and *skills* are implied in the role, many of which are described in Table 1.1. All of them are applied day-by-day according to experience, according to circumstances, and according to a changing pattern of requirements. Tables unfortunately cannot express movement, so the sense of frequent changes of scene is missing.

An important point to be made here about both the figure and the table is that they try to convey the idea that a manager cannot be adept at human relationships (i.e. good at dealing with people, be they doctors, nurses, clerical staff, or patients) without being conversant with the requisite procedures, forms, administrative systems, etc. which underpin good medical practice. The social skill which can defuse aggression shown by patients demanding instant

Table 1.1. *Tasks and responsibilities of the practice manager—some examples*

1. *People*
Doctors
    Organize rotas (right place at right time)
    Relieve them of administration
    Provide secretarial assistance
    Keep accurate diaries
    Hire locums
    Act as source of informal information
    Prepare trainee's programmes

Patients
    Organize clinics
    Respect confidentiality
    Ensure files up to date
    Know individual names and faces
    Listen to grumbles

Staff
    Interview and engage
    Know employment legislation
    Train newcomers
    Organize meetings
    Organize work rotas
    Encourage and motivate

2. *Finance*
    Keep accounts – budgets
    Balance books
    FPC returns – quarterly
    Item of service payments
    Salaries and wages
    PAYE and insurance
    Pay bills
    Car allowances
    Superannuation
    Petty cash
    Liaison with bank
    Cash flow (best time to purchase)

3. *Rules and procedures*
    Supervise appointments register
    Arrange holiday rotas
    Day book (messages)
    Phones – arrange night and weekend cover
    'Red Book' † – ensure best use made
    Age–sex register – keep up to date
    Filing – accuracy of patient data
    Mail – open and distribute
    Repeat prescriptions

4. *Building and stocks*
    Order supplies
    Check supplies regularly
    Purchase and maintain equipment (typewriters, photocopiers, etc.)
    Ensure security
    Housekeeping and cleaning
    Furniture and decoration
    Arrange maintenance and repairs
    Arrange adequate notice boards

Table 1.1.—*continued*

5. *Information*
   Visits and hospital discharges
   Births and deaths
   Policy changes – notify
   System for urgent messages
   Newsletter
   Patient handbook
   Prepare statistics
   Display notices, e.g. health education

6. *External agencies*
   FPC (Family Practitioner Committee)
   Hospitals and consultants
   District Health Authority
   Social Services (e.g. meals on wheels)
   Drug company representatives
   Community agencies, clubs, schools, etc.
   Pharmacists

† *Statement of Fees and Allowances.* DHSS. Issued to all GPs, and regularly updated.

attention is of limited practical use if at the same time the practice manager ignores the need for noticeboards, daybooks or other means to transmit important information. Other people have roles, too, which will be ineffective if they are left out of the script. Everyone with a part to play has to know the lines.

The balance

The practice manager has to achieve a delicate balance between the 'things' and the 'people', to act as the kind of linchpin implied by Fig. 1.1. Each segment, through the mediation of the practice manager, connects with the others. For example, any alteration to the appointments system (such as a decision to have more booked appointments) will affect people (doctors and administrative staff – everyone), space (waiting room usage), and external bodies (arrangements with the FPC). The manager will be expected, therefore, to anticipate the consequences of decisions reached by the practice and to ensure that the balance is not unduly tipped one way or another. To place emphasis upon procedural requirements above clinical decisions would be the wrong balance. The role presents a constant challenge to ingenuity. Table 1.1 sets out in more detail the principal tasks and responsibilities.

These are not intended to be comprehensive, all-inclusive lists but are drawn from analyses of their own jobs made by some 90 practice managers themselves,† and confirmed in other studies made of primary health-care teams in the Oxford Region (1978–9) and the Wessex Region (1980–1).

† At training courses for practice managers and senior staff run by the Royal College of General Practitioners (Thames Valley faculty) in conjunction with Oxford RHA, see Chapter 4.

Co-ordination

From what has been said so far it appears that the practice manager's primary task is to provide the link between activities and to help define priorities for the practice. Health care relies on: the professional and technical competence of trained people such as doctors and nurses; the patients' willingness to co-operate; and the efficient support of administrative systems. To make sure that all three are in harmony requires sensitive but firm skills of co-ordination.

An important function of a manager therefore is to act as a link between the doctors, the nurses, the health visitors, and so on on the one hand, and the clerical and reception staff on the other. She has to consider how far her responsibilities extend for the *co-ordination* of plans and of work for the medical and administrative staff alike. Words like planning and co-ordinating lack that sense of immediacy which characterizes most practices. They may seem remote from the reality of a practice manager's world, where the unspoken policy may be to deal with emergencies rather than to plan. However unless a manager is concerned with planning, she cannot expect to be able to co-ordinate the different and often disparate activities in general practice. A doctor may have to be pinned down, on a busy morning, to agree to do cervical smears on the one afternoon when Sister is available and when the majority of women in the age range are able to attend. At the same time, space is probably difficult to find so the clinic may have to be held somewhere different from normal. Time and effort are required to persuade, check back, ask someone to make the appointments, remind the doctor and Sister, and perhaps put up an additional notice. The practice manager can relieve the doctor, busy with his patients, from this need to co-ordinate simple but important activities.

Job descriptions cannot convey what this part of her work *feels* like, as nothing very tangible seems to result. The activity itself, such as the smear clinic, is not directly within the control of the person who has enabled it to take place, in other words who has co-ordinated the arrangements. This may explain why the desire to be in touch with real things and people is strong enough in most managers to make them want to take a turn in reception, to make the appointments, to answer patients' queries on the phone, to move the furniture around, fill in the forms, and so on. This is fine, so long as such activities do not become a substitute for the less tangible – and perhaps less immediately rewarding – responsibilities within a manager's role. To be busy in reception, in touch with people, can be more satisfying in the short term; meanwhile nobody is combing through the 'Red Book' to make certain the practice is making the best use of its facilities and skills to increase practice revenue.

Initiating

When a manager next feels impelled to be in the action at the front of the house, she might resist the temptation by sitting down (in the office, if she is lucky enough) to begin to make a list of *what* needs to be done, *when*, and by *whom.* The list would then be the agenda for a discussion at the next practice meeting and one would really have started to act like a manager, *initiating* as well as *planning*. In this way a pattern emerges of how the different tasks can fit together. One sees more than just details which have previously elicited an immediate response or decision. Priorities begin to emerge; some jobs can be delegated once they have been identified as being best done by someone other than the manager. A pattern evolves which makes sense because she has designed it. The textbooks on management use the word pro-active to describe this kind of management initiative. Another way to express the idea is the practice manager as leader, for hers is the principal leadership role amongst her own staff. She is in a position, because she plans and links activities together, to make sure that things happen.

Thinking about priorities

For many practice managers the scene described earlier will have been familiar with its instant demands, working against the clock, patients waiting anxiously, doctors busy in their rooms (sometimes, no doubt, uncertain themselves about their diagnoses) with barely enough time for the morning's crowded appointments. With all this happening around her the manager's problem was how to find time to be able to think clearly and to decide on priorities. She had to allocate to the different members of staff some of the innumerable jobs which had to be done, as well as decide what she must do herself. She had to persuade and cajole them into taking on some of the tasks – perhaps to tidy the bulky files. The tree needed attention too. And there was the trainee doctor, the absent staff member's sick pay, the fees and allowances, and so on. Determining priorities can so easily be postponed when you are faced with immediate pressures.

A surgery could be a much smarter, more efficiently run place were it not for having to take time to deal with patients – or at least a practice manager might be excused for thinking that! Although management of health care can seem to consist mainly of responding on the spur of the moment to a crisis or an emergency, time has to be found to work out what events take precedence. This is a manager's task even when doctors, under pressure, are demanding attention and the waiting room is bursting at its seams.

Job satisfaction can certainly be had through using one's skills and experience to deal with emergencies. At least there are tangible results. But if a busy practice is to function well, where full-time and part-time staff have different interlocking work rotas, then it has to be managed. Although the general practitioners are the business partners, it is not desirable for one of them to be the formal manager – they should be free to do the doctoring. Nevertheless they are a major influence upon the way the practice is managed, because of their stake in it. But they must understand what effective management can contribute and they must set up the framework in which the practice manager can give of her best. The doctor's role in management is considered in Chapter 7.

Taking stock

Time has to be made for someone to stand back from the hurly-burly to look at the kinds of demands being made on the staff. To do this 'thinking' part of the work is, admittedly, not easy and the inspiration to do so may come outside the surgery. Soaking in the bath or with one's feet up and the television turned off can be thinking occasions (why do we feel guilty at work if we put our feet up and try to reflect or plan, even if the waiting room is empty and the doctors are out on their visits?). But unless we can take stock of what is happening we are not likely to see the 'things', and the 'people' aspects of the practice as a complete picture. It will instead look like a random assortment of disconnected events. Reading this book might be one way for individual managers to begin to sort out their own role. There can be no ideal model, but there are ideas and experiences which can be thought about with advantage and related to each reader's particular circumstances. For the long-term effectiveness of a practice it may be more important to think ahead, as our manager did, about the over 75s category. She needed time to collect the facts and to put them to her doctors. Time for taking stock was therefore essential in the way she interpreted her role.

The art of management is to know which is the right choice to make between competing demands at any given moment, and therefore what is the most appropriate use of time and energy. The practice manager, as Fig. 1.1 implies, is engaged in a continuing balancing act between dealing with the immediate and making sure the future is also given some thought.

The need to manage the clinical and the administrative aspects of general practice has always been present. In the past the family doctor frequently employed, perhaps in an unofficial capacity, his wife who was nurse, receptionist, and bookkeeper. The practice was run from their home. Times have changed. The scope of general practice has widened, and extra responsibilities have been placed upon practices, some through legislation, such as the Employment Protection Act, in addition to the financial and tax obligations related to running a business. The requirements of a public health-care system, with its ever-changing structure, also create extra pressures upon doctors and their colleagues. The doctor now has many more specialists available to help his work, which gives emphasis to that vital co-ordinating function of the practice manager. These more recent developments merely underscore what, in fact, has always been so – the inescapable duty of people engaged in administering primary care to organize themselves and their work, varied as it is, in such a way as to ensure that the customers (the patients) receive proper treatment, help, and advice, and so can take more responsibility for their own health.

The relationship between doctor and patient is not the principal topic of this book, but in today's complex world with its changing social patterns, the maintenance of good health and the prevention of illness place different kinds of obligation upon patient and doctor alike. There, in the midst of all the activity, a 'bridge' between the practice and the general public, is the manager.

Managing a practice means being skilled in the four functions mentioned – planning, organizing, motivating, and evaluating – with a special emphasis on the art of co-ordinating and acting as intermediary. The manager as diplomat, perhaps?

Diplomat and mediator

So far we have looked at the kinds of work which a practice manager does either directly herself or through others for whom she has a managerial responsibility.

One group of managers, in attempting to summarize the essence of this role, saw it as being an intermediary – between patients and doctors; patients and staff; doctors and staff; and between the practice and the outside world of hospitals, social services, etc. Often it appeared to be a matter of 'smoothing troubled waters' or 'getting people together to sort out the middle areas'. In other words she is frequently the go-between, the mediator who provides a focus for everyone involved in health care at the primary level.

At times the possession of knowledge about the mechanics of her role, particularly the systems and procedures, is taken for granted. Most practice managers place emphasis upon the 'people' aspects of their work, not surprisingly where the care of patients is the dominant purpose. It would, however, be a dangerous assumption to believe that the 'things' do not require attention. New laws and new rules are introduced for the management of health care, so she must be up to date if they are to be correctly applied. However, from listening to managers and observing the kinds of activities in which they are involved, it appears that where they exercise most influence and where they feel they need most help, is in dealing with people. Medical care is about illness, accidents, even death and cannot be expected to create a uniformly relaxed atmosphere. Anxiety and tension will test everyone's tolerance and ability to get on with the job. Whilst such feelings may not be too difficult to cope with where subordinate colleagues are concerned, the solution is not so obvious when it involves doctors, other medical staff, or certain emotionally charged patients. Even an experienced practice manager can find that her hackles rise if the reception staff are having to face aggressive behaviour when this seems unwarranted. An ill-considered, hasty remark by a doctor on the spur of the moment can also create a tense atmosphere and the cool, calm practice manager's mediating influence is more than ever required. The practice manager, as Fig. 1.1 suggests, is at the centre of much of what happens.

The need for tolerance and sensitive understanding is particularly strong in her relationship with her colleagues, whose work is directly involved with patients, doctors, and nursing staff. She has no formal authority to exercise when dealing with medical staff; indeed, she may even be employed directly by the doctors whom she may see as being in a hierarchical position above her. She will still be expected to manage their workload so that the practice functions smoothly. The human aspects of managing a practice or health centre are not readily subject to rules and procedures, but they are an essential element within any practice manager's repertoire of skills.

THE PERSON

In Chapter 2 we consider the social skills which a manager needs. Before doing so we must recognize that the person, as well as the role, is a vital factor in any effective group. What kind of person might best be suited to this particular role of practice manager? Each manager, indeed each individual who works for the practice, will interpret her part in a unique way, dependent on different sets of experiences about medical practice in particular and about the world in general.

A manager may also be a housewife, mother, member of a church, the holder of political opinions, with her own views about society. As manager, therefore, she draws upon a range of experiences as well as being knowledgeable about rules and procedures essential to the running of the practice. Her qualities as a person will have been formed through a variety of experiences over her lifetime, as well as through more formal learning methods such as books, lectures, or courses. What might such a person be like, what are her characteristics, and how do these relate to the management of health care in the average practice?

Table 1.2 shows some of the attributes which a number of practice managers felt were important. The reader will be able to judge how closely such a description fits reality. Of course, no such paragon of virtue exists with all these estimable qualities; though it was the practice managers themselves who saw such qualities as desirable for their work. None the less, the list might serve as a guide for would-be practice managers as well as for experienced office-holders.

Table 1.2. *Personal qualities required by a practice manager (from statements made at the Oxford regional courses for practice managers)*

Adaptability	Responding to emergency but still keeping long-term plans in view.
Accessibility	Physically (not always in remote office) + psychologically (being receptive to others).
Diplomat	Smoothing the troubled waters.
Discretion	Asking the right questions, but not too bluntly.
Fairness-but-firmness	No favourites!
Humour	To defuse the tension.
Patience	Change does not happen overnight.
Persuasiveness	Able to convince with reason.
Self-awareness	Knowing what one does best and the limits of one's authority.
Tact	Not putting one's feet in!
Trust	Creating an atmosphere where others can be open, by being open oneself.
Unflappability	Counting to ten, even when things are hectic. Doing several jobs simultaneously.

2 Staff

The last two decades have seen major changes in the way general practice is conducted, and one important change has been in the employment of more staff to help the doctor by taking over administrative and nursing tasks.

The *Statement of fees and allowances* (the 'Red Book') states that the reimbursement scheme applies to staff directly employed by the doctor or partnership, excluding wives and families of the doctors, although in the last few years this exclusion has been relaxed and it is now possible for an allowance to be claimed by a single-handed general practitioner receiving either rural practice allowance or inducement payment in respect of his wife or dependent relative who is working on a regular basis of at least 19 hour per week.

Any general practitioner who is in receipt of a basic practice allowance automatically becomes eligible for reimbursement of staff. Staff will qualify only if engaged in one or more of the following duties:

(1) secretarial and clerical work (including records);
(2) reception of patients;
(3) making appointments;
(4) dispensing;
(5) nursing and treatment.

A member of staff must work a minimum of five hours per week and the doctor may claim up to two whole-time equivalent staff per doctor (whole time being recognized as a 38 hour week).

There is still tremendous scope for employment of staff, since on average each general practitioner employs just a little over one whole-time equivalent staff member. Each doctor must ask himself 'Am I employing the optimum number of staff?' 'Could I work more effectively with more staff, and thereby free myself of administrative duties in order to improve patient care, the organization of the practice, or just have a better life?'

Employing practice staff is one of the most difficult tasks that the practice manager, either herself, or in conjunction with the doctors, will have to undertake. Unfortunately there is no magic formula and it would be foolhardy to state that, if you follow the rules, all will go well; however, it is possible to offer guidelines and to pinpoint some of the pitfalls.

There is quite a range of titles given by doctors to staff and in the main these are: receptionists, secretaries, shorthand-typists, audio-typists, filing clerks,

clerks, administrative secretaries, and practice managers. However, as is often the case, the receptionist in one practice may be called the medical secretary in another; the practice manager in one, the senior secretary in another. It is therefore not the name that is important, but more the allocation of duties. If one thinks of the general practice office workload under three main categories: reception, secretarial, and administrative, the appropriate title for the post will inevitably fall into place.

The very atmosphere of the practice depends upon the reception that the patient receives when presenting at the desk. This underlines the importance of the receptionist's job, and the care needed in her selection and training. The 'Let's advertise and see who turns up' approach will most certainly lead to trouble and employing a new member of staff should have its beginning long before this.

Step 1: assess the needs

The post offered will need to be thoroughly analysed, thinking through exactly what is required, jotting down notes, and discussing ideas and suggestions with other members of staff until a clear job description emerges. When a vacancy arises it may well be appropriate to hold a practice doctor/staff meeting to decide if changes are needed in the allocation of work, rather than automatically replacing staff.

Step 2: job description

This popular phrase sounds most formal, but is no more than a clear idea of what the employer requires from the proposed new member of staff; her duties and tasks listed on paper for ease of reference and understanding amongst colleagues. No two practices are alike, which makes general practice so diverse and exciting, so the following job descriptions for a medical receptionist and medical secretary must be seen only as a guide.

Medical receptionist: a person of first contact for the patient – either by telephone, or personal contact.

1. Receive patients in reception area, noting their attendance on appointment sheet, or making appointments as requested.
2. Provide patients with information as required.
3. Receive incoming calls, recording messages accurately in the form as agreed by the practice, and transfer calls as appropriate to health visitor, doctor, nurse, etc.
4. Oversee and supervise waiting area.
5. Extract patients records in advance of consultation sessions.
6. Maintain all clerical aspects of repeat prescription service.
7. File records following consultations.
8. File hospital mail for Dr – and Dr –.

9. Tidy desks in consulting rooms, checking full range of forms and re-stocking as appropriate.

10. Chaperone patients as requested.

11. Report to colleague taking over reception duty, on any issue not complete, e.g. request for home visit not passed on to the doctor.

Medical secretary

1. Open all incoming mail and distribute to the person who will be dealing with it.

2. Type all outgoing letters, always ensuring copy for patient's records.

3. Type all forms and other papers relating to patients, or financial claims for item of service treatment.

4. Keep diary.

5. Make travel arrangements for doctors attending post-graduate courses.

6. Record data for at-risk register (such as diabetic register).

7. Record data for hypertension screening and recall system.

8. Supervise stocks and order all practice stationery.

9. Cover receptionist's duties over the lunchtime period, 1 p.m.–2 p.m. daily and at other times if required.

10. Collate statistics into tables month by month (home visits, consultations, and hospital referrals).

11. Post mail daily.

12. Purchase stamps and record. Balance book monthly.

13. Petty cash – record. Balance book monthly.

In a smaller general practice where there is no administrative secretary or practice manager, the doctor would have to consider delegating the supervision of such administrative duties as arranging a gardener, window cleaner, cleaning of the premises, etc., to the senior receptionist.

Step 3: specification

Having completed the job description, it is now time to think about a written specification of the type of person you wish to employ for this vacancy, which by now is a clearly defined role: age, experience, special skills, personal attributes – the latter being particularly important and often the most difficult to assess. This step makes it easier to match applicants against the requirements of the job, and against each other. It introduces some system into a field where people can easily be swayed by personal preferences.

Step 4: staff salaries

A salary scale which is fair, pays the correct rate for the job, and is consistent is absolutely essential to ensure high morale and good working relations. Sorting out staff salaries fairly may be difficult because of the different job titles and duties. Staff, quite naturally, talk to their colleagues within and outside their own particular place of work and soon realize that great disparities exist.

By far the most fair method is to obtain a copy of the Whitley Council gradings for public employees in the National Health Service, which contains a table which gives the annual salary and hourly rate for each job (e.g. receptionist, shorthand typist), according to age. These rates are based on hospital and office work with much less stress and responsibility than that in general practice, and should be regarded as a minimum. In addition, general-practice staff work unsocial hours for which overtime rates cannot be reimbursed, so this factor must be incorporated in the basic rate.

The following people and professional bodies also give helpful information on national scales (addresses in Appendix F):

The Association of Medical Secretaries, Practice Administrators and Receptionists;
The Association of Health Centre and Practice Administrators;
The Information Resources Centre, RCGP.
The Finance Officer of the Family Practitioner Committee (Health Board in Scotland);
The Personnel Officer of the health authority or board.

Such a scale can be used as a basis, but varied to take account of special factors such as additional skills and responsibilities. Salaries must be seen to be based on the correct rate for the job. The incremental points must be clearly stated. Fairness and consistency must be the aim at all times. Scales are also published regularly in *Pulse, Medeconomics,* and *General Practitioner.*

At this stage the practice manager will know exactly what tasks have to be covered, the type of person they wish to employ to undertake the tasks, and the salary scale and conditions of service. The next stage is to advertise the vacancy.

A note of caution: it is often at this point that the doctor knows just the right person 'Mrs Smith, down the road, recently widowed, a little depressed, only a few days ago told me she feels that a job would get her out and about again and I do agree that it would be good for her!' The doctor, by the very nature of his profession, looks after his patient's emotional well-being and does indeed know what is good for her – but not necessarily and automatically 'good' for the overall smooth running of the practice.

Step 5: advertising and informing

The advertisement can now be prepared and placed in the local newspaper. Some newspapers have particularly appropriate nights for 'job vacancies', special rates for more than one insertion, straight column, semi-display advertising, etc. Normally a very efficient sales person in the 'tele-ads' office of the newspaper will be able to help, but remember that advertising is expensive and sales talk may need to be resisted!

The purpose of the advertisement is both to attract applicants, and to allow them to decide at an early stage if they match the main requirements of the post. So the advertisement should be explicit and be based on the job description and specification. Details of hours of work required, for example, would avoid interviewing applicants where such hours were totally unsuitable.

An advertisement for a receptionist may read:

Receptionist required for busy general medical practice in south of city. Hours 8.30 a.m.–2 p.m. Mon.–Fri. Alternate Sat. 8.30 a.m.–1 p.m. Apply in own handwriting to Box No. − with the names of two references.

Some practices prefer to use box numbers since patients may notice the vacancy advertised with *their* doctor's practice, and duly make an appointment to see him, thereby attempting to by-pass the correct process of applying for the post. The doctor may find this situation, because of his relationship with the patient, rather difficult and embarrassing. Box numbers are efficient and redirect applications by first-class post as they arrive. A small charge is made for this facility, in addition to the basic advertisement charge. Not all practices need the barrier of a box number, and are prepared to give their name, address, and telephone number. This provides a direct and personal link which may better reflect the philosophy of the practice.

Ten years ago one would have expected in a city practice to receive perhaps six or seven applications for such a post. In these difficult days of high unemployment one may expect to receive even hundreds of applications, including many from school leavers.

An alternative to advertising the vacancy would be to contact a local College of Further Education or Polytechnic which runs specific courses for the training of medical secretaries and medical receptionists. A secretarial agency is another source of staff, particularly if time is short.

It is quite customary for the job description and other details such as holiday entitlement, sick pay, and hours of duty to be sent to all applicants. The individual then has the opportunity of assessing her own suitability and ability for the post and may withdraw the application at this early stage if it would be sensible to do so. In sending information to the applicant, and in the way the application is handled, the practice is revealing the way it works. Selecting staff is a two-way process. They too can choose or reject the opportunity.

Step 6: short listing

If a large number of applications is received, short-listing is necessary and the practice manager may undertake this in total, or may read all applications, noting down short comments, based on a comparison of the application with the job specification. The comments would be passed to the doctors, or to the doctor charged with responsibility to assist. Such observations would include:

general appearance and neatness of letter;
educational standard, and special aptitudes;
experience;
age;
commitments.

Applications usually fall into three categories:

(1) most suitable;
(2) possibly suitable;
(3) definitely *not* suitable.

Between five and ten applicants can be short-listed. If there are only two or three applicants it is wise to see them all, even if they are personally known. An interview may reveal unsuspected problems, or bonus points.

Step 7: interviewing and deciding

Initial interviews may be undertaken by the practice manager on her own, but it is wiser for two people to be involved if selection and rejection are taking place. Not only are two heads better than one, but they give protection against charges of unfair discrimination. Interviews may be conducted by the practice manager, one of the doctors, or in the case of health authority employees, by the personnel officer or manager concerned.

The setting for the interview should be as relaxed and informal as possible; sitting round a room or round a table is better than facing the candidate across a desk. Everyone should be able to see one another, so no-one should have a bright window behind them.

Notes are best written after an interview, so time must be allowed for this. An opportunity should be found for candidates to meet other members of staff, and see round the premises. Some of the candidates may be unable to take time off work for interviews, so flexible arrangements are essential if good applicants are not going to be lost.

A proforma for all the available details of the candidate may be helpful as a check list, so that data are not missing. As well as name, address, telephone number, date of birth, and civil status, headings could cover such information as:

educational attainments/qualifications;
past experience;
present health;
outside commitments/interests;
holidays already arranged;
when free to start if appointed.

Making rational choices between candidates is difficult. It can be made more objective by considering it according to a schedule such as Rodger's 'Seven-point plan', which would cover the following questions.

1. *Physical make-up*
   Is the candidate's health and physique adequate for the job? Are his or her appearance, bearing, and speech agreeable?
2. *Attainments*
   What type of education has the candidate had, and what standards have been achieved? What occupational training and experience has she had?
3. *General intelligence*
   How much general intelligence can, or does the candidate display?
4. *Special aptitudes*
   Has the candidate any special skills or aptitudes relevant to the job?
5. *Interests*
   What practical, social, artistic, or other interests does the candidate have?
6. *Disposition*
   How acceptable is the candidate to other people? Is she able to influence others, dependable, and self-reliant?
7. *Circumstances*
   What are the domestic circumstances of the candidate in so far as they may be relevant to the job?

Using the job specification, and some of the seven points listed above, it may be possible to draw up a list of essential qualities needed for the job, and another list of desirable qualities. Each selector can draw up a score card as in Table 2.1.

Table 2.1. *Score card for selection interviews*

	Candidate			
Essential qualities (score 1–5)	A	B	C	D
'Essential' Total				
Desirable qualities (score 1–5)				
'Desirable' Total				

This method is a useful aid to a decision between candidates who seem equally acceptable. It may help to make the process of choice more systematic, but it still depends on the subjective judgement of the selector. Each candidate can be compared on essential qualities, and if a decision is not clear, then desirable qualities can be taken into consideration. The candidates interviewed should be listed in order of acceptability, not just one chosen.

References should be taken up before the selection interview. Written references are less satisfactory than the names and addresses of referees who can be approached in confidence about the applicant's suitability. Referees can be more frank over the telephone than on paper, when the general tone is bland, and failings are glossed over.

Some applicants are embarrassed to give the name of their current employer as a referee unless they get the job, as it makes it clear that the employee is thinking of leaving. In such cases the references can be taken up after the post is offered 'subject to references'.

Travelling expenses of all applicants interviewed should be paid without question.

Step 8: notifying the successful applicant

The successful applicant must be told as soon as possible, perhaps immediately after completion of interviews, or by telephone, but this verbal notification must be followed up by a formal letter from the practice, offering the post and requesting that she replies in writing indicating acceptance.

Step 9: notifying the unsuccessful applicants

The other candidates interviewed should not be rejected until the one at the top of the list has accepted. They should each receive a personal letter to thank them for applying. Other applicants should be notified that the post has been filled. If there have been many applications, a photocopied letter would suffice.

Further guidance can be found in:

Management check lists. No. 8 *Filling a vacancy* and No. 9 *Selecting staff*, published by the British Institute of Management, Parker Street, London WC2B 5PT.

Selection interviewing, (1982) by Peter Whitaker. The Industrial Society, 3 Carlton House Terrace, London SW1Y 5DG.

Guide to employment practices (1983) by Betty Ream, also published by the Industrial Society.

The Seven Point Plan, by (the late) Professor Alec Rodger. Paper No. 1. 3rd Edn. 1970. NFER-Nelson Publishing, Windsor, Berks.

Just as the advertisement is not the first step when employing staff, so the step of 'post offered and accepted' is not the end.

Step 10: legal responsibilities and liabilities

The employment law is complex and concerned principally with large-scale business. The general practitioner, in keeping with any other employer in the country must look to his legal responsibilities. In the last few years employment law has undergone radical changes. The law stipulates the rights and obligations of both employer and employee, and must be known and understood. The general practitioner who refuses to accept his responsibilities as an employer may be paving the way for endless problems. If, however, he is prepared to understand the basic requirements of the law and to take his responsibilities as an employer seriously and work as a team with his staff, he is unlikely to encounter legal difficulties or problems. It would be unreasonable to expect a general practitioner to understand all the employment law but some important areas are outlined below, in which the practice manager can assist.

Sex and race discrimination

People should be selected solely on their ability to do the job, with no discrimination allowed on the grounds of sex or race. For example, the Sex Discrimination Act of 1975 states that an advertisement must not specify the sex of the applicant.

Contract of employment

By the thirteenth week of employment, provided the employee works 16 hours per week or over, the Employment Protection (Consolidation) Act of 1978 states that the employer has to give the employee a written Contract of Employment.

A contract exists from the moment a post is offered verbally. After acceptance it may be strengthened by an exchange of letters, although doctors often neglect to give a written contract. This may be due to the friendly and personal relationship between the doctor and staff so that the introduction of legal papers might be seen as an unnecessary intrusion. If the practice manager can show that the Contract of Employment (like the job description) is merely the setting down of agreements and understandings about the post, the contract will be seen to be sensible and far less formidable than the term implies.

The contract should contain the following:

(1) name of parties to be contracted;
(2) title of the post held;
(3) details of pay scale with incremental dates clearly indicated;
(4) sick pay;
(5) when and how employee is to be paid;
(6) place of work;
(7) hours of work;
(8) holidays entitlement (including arrangements for public holidays);
(9) service days (extra days off for long service);
(10) pension details – if any;
(11) length of notice;
(12) grievance procedure;
(13) health and safety at work;
(14) wearing of uniform and name badge;
(15) breach of confidentiality leading to dismissal.

The practice manager may wish to draw up her own form for use as a contract of employment but contract forms are available from a number of sources, such as business stationers. The BMA regional offices offer assistance to BMA members on such issues as contracts of employment and how to introduce the written contract among ancillary staff. Many general practitioners have already made use of the contract of employment form issued from this source. Alternatively the Health Authority personnel officer may provide a copy of the official form.

Holidays

Holidays are not statutory entitlements, but are agreed mutually. A full-time member of staff would be expected to receive at least four weeks annual holidays, stating that in the main, one week should be taken in the period from March to May, two weeks in the period from June to September, etc., or whatever appears compatible to the needs of the practice. There may also be a proviso that not more than two staff members take their holidays at the same time without special consent.

Sickness

Sickness benefit became an employee's statutory right in 1983 when the Social Security and Housing Benefits Act came into force. The employer became the paymaster, and is responsible for the payment of eligible employee's benefit for up to eight weeks' sick leave in a tax year. For further details see Ellis (1983).

Service days

A service-days scheme is in operation in many large businesses and can quite easily be adapted to the general practice setting. Awarding service days is one way of simply saying 'thank you' to a member of staff who has been loyal and worked with the practice for perhaps 10 years, whilst her colleague of four years' service has now reached parity on the pay scale.

Staff pensions

There was a brief period up to February 1978 when staff pension contributions qualified for reimbursement. Now they do not, so the practice must bear the cost less income tax. There is an alternative, which has been well described in Money Pulse (7 August 1982).† Under this scheme staff members are paid an additional salary, to compensate for the lack of pension, on the understanding that they will use this as a contribution to a pension scheme. The practice gets 70 per cent reimbursement and tax relief. The staff member receives tax relief on pension contributions. However, there is no compulsion on the staff member to use the extra salary for pension contributions. This seems a fair way

---

†Further details are available from Michael Turner, Pulse Insurance Bureau, 147 Connaught Avenue, Frinton-on-Sea, Essex.

of recognizing that Whitley scales, which include an index-linked pension, are not an adequate basis for the salary of staff who are not pensionable. Staff employed by health authorities have full pension rights, and it will not be long before non-pensioned staff feel they are losing out.

When one considers that the employer's contributions to a pension scheme are tax deductible and that many members of staff work in a full-time capacity and have every intention of making a career in general practice, such members of staff could expect the provision of a pension. Various insurance brokers offer extremely attractive pension plans. In some practices the GP has discussed the provision of a pension with members of staff and agreed mutually that it would be more profitable to forgo an increment in salary and take a larger pension. The contract of employment shows details of the pension scheme in operation: the name of the scheme and the benefits that it offers.

The length of notice

Unlike holidays and sick pay, where practice policy prevails, the length of notice that an employee can expect is governed by the ruling as laid down in the 1978 Employment Protection (Consolidation) Act. The minimum requirements are that one week's notice is required if the employee has worked more than four weeks but less than two years. Each additional year worked warrants a further week's notice, with the maximum being set at 12 years, which would be 12 week's notice. It is worthwhile noting that these are minimum requirements and that it is generally accepted that a member of staff on monthly salary would receive a month's notice. It is the responsibility of the individual practice to write into the contract exactly what is required to allow ample time for finding a replacement.

Redundancy rights

In years past the term 'redundancy payment' was heard of only when a person's job ceased to exist in total because a firm or company went out of business altogether. The redundancy rights as laid down in the Redundancy Payments Act covers a wider range of situations over and above this original interpretation. An employee would have grounds to claim redundancy payment if:

1. Their job ceased to exist.

Example: An elderly general practitioner retiring with a small list size, the practice being disbanded, and the patients being allocated to other general practitioners in the area.

2. Their job is no longer required for financial or other reason.

Example: Installation of a computer to improve the records system enabling one person to handle the data input, instead of two presently employed to look after the manual system.

3. Their place of work is being changed to the extent that it would not be possible, or would be difficult, for the employee to continue their job of work.

Example: A practice closing its premises completely and moving some considerable distance to join with an existing group, or health centre.

It is difficult to be precise on redundancy rights and the above is given as guidance only. Individual cases in dispute would be looked at by a tribunal who would determine what is a reasonable request and what is not.

It is therefore important that the practice manager considers at an early stage exactly what it will mean to members of staff when discussing improving the organization, or a move to new premises, etc. For example, if a doctor moves premises and this involves a change in the condition of the job, he must make the employee an offer of the new post within a period of four weeks from the expiry of the old one. If the post offered is reasonably similar to the old post and the distance to travel marginally further than to the old premises, then the employee would probably be unable to claim redundancy payment. The employee has a period of four weeks in which to decide whether the new place of work and conditions are suitable. If not to her liking the employee may resign and not lose the right to take up a claim for redundancy payment.

In all examples of redundancy mentioned, if the practice is in a position to make the employee an offer of new employment that is reasonable and makes the offer within the prescribed period of four weeks from the expiry of the old position, it is more than likely that the right to redundancy payment will be lost.

Complaints procedure

It is a requirement that a complaints or grievance procedure is established so that the employee has a written statement of the procedure to follow if dissatisfied, or in conflict with disciplinary action. Unfair dismissals leading to industial tribunals are all too common, though thankfully very rarely heard of in the general practice setting. None the less (as has been demonstrated throughout this chapter), the wise practice will write down this procedure as an integral part of the contract document, or annexed to it.

Misconduct

Discipline would be the logical action following misconduct and the employee should be informed exactly what action the employer (or the person responsible for staff) would take in such circumstances, and indeed clearly what would be termed misconduct. Theft would most definitely warrant disciplinary action, as would a breach of confidentiality such as a receptionist discussing a patient's medical record information with a third party. The two examples given would in many instances warrant instant dismissal, although the practice manager or general practitioner would have to be absolutely certain of the facts and be in no doubt that the employee had been guilty of such gross misconduct. Discipline and eventual dismissal of an employee is a serious business. It may be helpful to bear in mind the ACAS Code of Practice, at least the essential elements of the code as they would relate to the general-practice setting. ACAS† is the Advisory Conciliation and Arbitration Service (the Government body charged with promoting harmonious relations between employees and employers).

Points to remember:

1. Always make it absolutely clear to members of staff what rules apply to their particular posts or general-practice policy, e.g. smoking, wearing of uniform, confidentiality, stealing.

2. Make it known what action would follow if the rules are broken.

3. Consider separately individual instances of misconduct not specifically set down.

4. Keep written records.

Trades unions and professional associations

NALGO, COHSE, and NUPE are the three most common unions appropriate to doctor's ancillary staff. Many practices throughout the country employ a practice nurse who should be encouraged to be a member of the Royal College of Nursing and to use their liability insurance. The practice may be wise to undertake the payment of the annual subscription on behalf of the practice nurse.

Health and safety

The doctor (as any other employer) has to note the Health and Safety at Work Act, whereby he is responsible for adequate measures to be taken to ensure the health and safety of those in his employment.

Health and safety legislation lays down minimum standards to ensure that the working population of the country is protected, and accidents prevented when possible. Whilst the legislation is of particular importance for factories and other industrial settings, the law states that an employer is bound to provide adequate heat and light, ventilation, toilets, and washing facilities and also to take adequate steps to ensure that members of staff will not be injured by faulty equipment – such as a dangerous frayed cable on electrical equipment, insecure filing cabinets, broken areas of floor-covering causing an uneven surface, unstable furniture. An important part of the practice manager's job will be the maintenance of equipment and premises.

Whilst the overall responsibility for health and safety at work rests with the employer, the practice manager would wish to encourage all members of staff to realize that they too have a legal duty to take reasonable care to avoid injury, with particular respect to medical instruments, prams, and so on. Any accident to a member of staff or to a member of the public should be reported immediately to the doctor or practice manager, who should record the full details of all the circumstances relating to the accident.

The reader may by now feel the great weight of responsibility that an employer incurs, so it may be reassuring to include here the final paragraph of an article

†ACAS: Clifton House, Euston Road, London, NW1 2RS.

written by Norman Ellis, Under-Secretary and Senior Industrial Relations Officer with the BMA on the Employment Law:

In my experience many of the problems of general practitioners are caused by poor selection procedures when staff are first appointed, inadequate supervision, and a reluctance to act decisively when staff are found to be unsatisfactory. Of course, for the general practitioner who employs only a few staff it is pointless to recommend formal procedures drawn from the practices of large organisations for the recruitment, appointment, and discipline of staff. The best advice that can be offered is that basic commonsense principles should be applied to these matters. The general practitioners should take great care to recruit the right staff, they should serve a probationary period with effective procedures for assessing their performance, and the general practitioner should not hesitate to take firm action if their performance fails to meet the standard required.

The legislation likely to affect employees of general practitioners is given in Table 2.2. This is a brief summary of a complex subject, and should be regarded as a guide rather than an authoritative source; the references quoted should be consulted when in doubt.

Further reading on employed staff

Ellis, N. (1987). *Employing staff,* 2nd Edn. British Medical Association. This booklet contains a series of articles from the British Medical Journal by one of its under-secretaries who is an expert in this field. It covers a wide range of topics, and includes the latest legislation on employment and statutory sick pay. Every practice manager should read this book, and have it handy for reference.

The Industrial Society. A series of booklets on subjects related to employment are available from the society at a very modest cost. Publications catalogue available on request from: The Industrial Society, Freepost, London SW1Y 5BR. Also from regional offices. The titles available are listed in Appendix G (page 274). *Guide to employment practices,* and *Selection interviewing* are useful.

British Institute of Management. Management checklists are published on a wide variety of topics, including filling a vacancy, and selecting staff. Apply to B.I.M., Management House, Parker Street, London WC2B 5PT.

Video Arts Ltd. have some excellent booklets, films and videos on staff management, for example on selection interviewing, appraisal interviews and communication. (For address see p. 273).

LOCUM GENERAL PRACTITIONERS

Many group practices can cover holiday relief and post-graduate training without employing a locum. But when a partner falls ill, a locum may be needed in a hurry.

Holiday cover puts an extra strain on busy partners, so many practices now use locums. If regular arrangements can be made, the locum gets to know the practice policies as well as many of the patients, who are less reluctant to see a familiar locum.

Table 2.2. *Summary of legislation affecting the employees of general practitioners*

Who is eligible	Legislation
Any applicant for job	
Not to be discriminated against on the grounds of marriage or sex	Sex Discrimination Act 1975
Not to be discriminated against on the grounds of colour, race, nationality, or ethnic, or national origins	Race Relations Act 1976
Any employee	
To receive equal pay with a member of the opposite sex doing similar work	Equal Pay Act 1970
Not to have action taken against him/her because of trade union membership or activity	Employment Protection (Consolidation) Act 1978
To have time off for certain trade union activities, unpaid though in some circumstances employee is entitled to paid time off	Employment Protection (Consolidation) Act 1978
To have time off for public duties – e.g. jury service	Employment Protection (Consolidation) Act 1978
To receive an itemized pay statement	Employment Protection (Consolidation) Act 1978
To have paid time off for ante natal care	Employment Act 1980
To receive sick pay for up to 28 weeks of sickness absence in a tax year, though in some circumstances there is no right to sick pay	Social Security and Housing Benefits Act 1982, as amended 1985
Any employee working 16 hours or more a week (after five years' employment any employee working eight hours or more)	
To be given a minimum period of notice – based on length of service – termination of employment	Employment Protection (Consolidation) Act 1978
Any employee with at least 13 weeks' service (five years service if employee works more than eight hours per week but less than 16 hours)	
To receive a written statement of terms of employment	Employment Protection (Consolidation) Act 1978
Any employee with at least 104 weeks service	
Not to be unfairly dismissed	Employment Protection (Consolidation) Act 1978 and Employment Act 1980, as amended 1985
Not to be dismissed on grounds of pregnancy Employees working 8 to 16 hours per week the period of eligibility becomes 5 years	Employment protection (Consolidation) Act 1978, as amended 1985

(Table cont. overleaf)

Table 2:2—*continued*

Who is eligible	Legislation
Any employee with at least 104 weeks service (cont.)	
To receive maternity pay and return to work up to 29 weeks after birth of child, but only if continuously employed until 11th week before expected date of deliver, for emploees working more than 16 hours per week. For employees who work 8 to 16 hours per week the eligibility becomes 5 years	Employment Protection (Consolidation) Act 1978
To return to work after absence due to pregnancy – same kind of job in the same place and same capacity.	
To have time off, with pay, to seek alternative work or to arrange training if made redundant.	Employment Protection (Consolidation) Act 1978

The practice manager has an important part to play – initially in encouraging the partners to decide well in advance whether a locum is needed. She can then consult her 'locum book' in which she keeps names, addresses, telephone numbers, and availability of locums. The pool of locums is constantly changing and only by keeping in touch with the vocational training course, her colleagues in other practices, and the FPC administrator can she keep the locum book up to date. If this method fails, she may have to resort to advertisements (free in some of the give-away medical journals), contacting the British Medical Association Personal Services Bureau† (locum section), or local BMA office.

If the locum is not well-known to the practice, a check should be made that he is registered. In all cases, the locum should be covered by insurance against professional negligence or malpractice. In spite of this the employing partner(s) is responsible for the treatment of his patients by the locum, who should therefore be chosen with care.

It should be made clear whether the locum is doing a set surgery (e.g. 9.00–11 a.m., 4.00–6.00 p.m.) or an open-ended one, with or without visits. Normally the locum would provide his own diagnostic instruments and car.

If the locum is to cover obstetrics, then a check should be made that this is acceptable to the FPC. The FPC should, in any case, be informed of holiday and locum arrangements.

Fees and mileage rates should be agreed beforehand. The BMA personal services bureau publishes a list of average charges, but this is not a rigid scale of fees. However most practices pay 'BMA rates'. *Medeconomics* publishes the rates regularly. Mileage is usually paid from home to home.

HUMAN RELATIONSHIPS AND INDIVIDUAL SOCIAL SKILLS

For work to be done there has to be give and take between people, who may not always see eye to eye. We are all different from each other to some degree,

† BMA House, Tavistock Square, London, WC1H 9JP. Telephone: 01-387-0611.

through social, educational, or physical circumstances. It is inevitable that we will have different perceptions of *what* has to be achieved and even greater ones about *how* to do it. We do not necessarily share the same goals – managers may wish to change working arrangements to gain greater efficiency, while other staff may have shorter-term aims to protect their own interests. From time to time disputes arise, occasionally leading to bitter conflict.

Sensitivity towards people

In health care, there can be no fundamental disagreement about what people are employed to do, because of daily reminders in the form of patients and persistent telephone calls. A difference in emphasis there may well be, between those who wish to concentrate on prevention of ill-health or injury, and those who see their chief function as responding to demand from patients, and helping them to cope with everyday life. Whatever the differences about priorities and especially about the allocation of resources, *people*, with their whims and foibles are a continuing factor. Whether one is a doctor, nurse, receptionist, secretary, or practice manager, an understanding about what motivates people to behave as they do is essential. For the practice manager this means the development and application of sensitivity towards colleagues and patients in order to provide more effective administrative support to the primary task – the provision of health care. The study and practice of human relations goes beyond 'being nice to people on company time' (Whyte 1956). It means being aware of a number of different factors which influence attitudes, and trying to understand behaviour as it relates to specific tasks and to specific contexts. Sensitivity is a first requisite. The skills which flow from this are acquired through practice.

Staff morale has to be one of the manager's first considerations. As with patient morale, this derives from mutual respect and tolerance. Respect for her authority is based on a recognition by others of her competence. The most obvious sign of this competence is the degree of awareness which she shows to the needs of people, both staff and patients. In health care, urgent demands are sometimes made on people who may already be overloaded with work, so it is essential to convey a sense that the right hand *does* know what the left hand is doing. The manager, must ensure that there is:

confidence in the professional competence of staff;
respect for individuals, including patients;
cohesive team work, making a reality of an integrated unit.

Awareness and sensitivity to colleagues, patients, and one's surroundings are fundamental attributes for a manager who wishes to combine administrative skills with those of managing people. A good manager must take account of the background factors against which a practice develops its policy. For example, the problems of a single-handed rural practice will differ from those of an inner-city practice. The latter might have to cope with dilapidated premises; the former with inadequate public transport for patients. The social skills of a practice manager will ensure that she can respond to environmental influences like these, as well as to procedural tasks, such as organizing team meetings, running a series of clinics, communicating with hospitals, and so on. Different emphasis will be placed on different skills according to circumstances.

Custom and practice

Most of us learn to understand the behaviour of others, and to adapt to it where necessary. As we develop and grow so we learn how to behave, in more senses than one. To use a jargon phrase we become 'socialized'. In other words we learn to survive and make progress as members of the various groups we join. We learn the rules, the taboos, and the norms which people establish in order to achieve particular aims. We know which rules we have to comply with, which we break at our peril, and which we can test out to see if we can modify. The practice manager soon becomes aware of the norms of the practice which help it to function. Norms should not be thought of as good or bad, but as part of the general fabric which expresses that unique feel of a place. A manager would wish to suggest changes only after a careful consideration of how they might affect the functioning of the place as a whole. Sensitivity to human behaviour, particularly at work, teaches us that most resistance to change or rejection of new proposals occurs when these unofficial rules or norms are threatened.

A newly appointed manager begins her job by observing and listening, and noting what seem to be the general style of the practice. To rush in with bright ideas about drastic changes, even over relatively simple arrangements ('as from next Monday there will be no coffee break but staff will take a break in relays') would indicate a lack of social skill, and certainly of a basic sensitivity. Not a very helpful approach to the management of people engaged in health care.

Responsibilities involving people

The managers who attended two Oxford Region Courses in 1980 (referred to in Chapter 1) listed the activities to which they felt most time was devoted. According to their estimates about half their time was taken up with paperwork, and half with what was loosely called 'dealing with people'. This included:

(1) Staff management, i.e. those people directly responsible to the practice manager;
(2) Patient management;
(3) Employment, and termination of employment of staff;
(4) Co-ordination between doctors and other staff.

Although each practice or centre has its own unique character, many of the skills required to manage will be common. The four areas of 'people' responsibilities considered as being important by managers themselves contain two broad categories of skills, those related to individuals and those related to groups. These categories are not intended to be mutually exclusive, although communication face-to-face between two people is of a different kind from that involved in leading a group discussion where the views of a number of disciplines represented in the practice are expressed. (Communications between people in groups will be dealt with in Chapter 3).

Let us now consider in what ways a practice manager is likely to find herself involved with a single individual during the course of a typical day's work. Relationships at work between individual people depend on a number of factors, according to whether the relationship is based on formal roles, e.g. doctor to practice manager, receptionist to patient, or whether it is a colleague relationship as between friends who know each other socially; or it may be a mixture of both.

For a manager, then, it is important to understand her role within the different contexts where she deals with individuals at work. She may have to rebuke a part-time clerk who keeps arriving late, but she does so in her role as manager. She may have to act as an informal, unofficial sounding board for one of the doctors keen to try out new ideas about manning the surgery (the skill of listening is as vital as the skill of telling). She may find herself being a wise 'mother' to an anxious young health visitor who is wary of the rather formidable senior partner. Whatever her roles, formal or informal, and they may not be listed amongst the duties in her job description, the manager's skills must ensure that her colleagues do not become confused by her failure to distinguish between them. She will have to handle sensitively the information to which she is privy as a patient's friend for example, even when tempted to use the information when wearing her official hat, as chairman of the weekly meeting.

The emphasis so far has been upon the importance for a practice manager to develop a sense of awareness which can lead to insights about behaviour of people. We will now examine how these insights can be of practical use in her everyday contacts with patients, doctors, staff, and the people with whom she has to deal in the world beyond the practice.

Interviewing skills and techniques

One activity which every manager undertakes is the conduct of face-to-face discussions, whether this be a formal interview to determine an applicant's suitability, for example, or an informal chat with one of her colleagues who is seeking advice. The purpose may differ, but the skills required in this kind of two-way communication are similar. After all, whatever the situation, two people are trying to convey by word and by gesture what they think and feel, even if their objectives differ. The process of interviewing cannot be a mechanistic procedure with a rigid set of rules to cover every occasion. Simple guidelines will help; practice alone will develop the skill. The principal guidelines are as follows.

Clarity of objective

The manager, as the person who either sets up the interview or responds to another's request, must be clear from the outset what she intends to be the outcome. If the objective is clear in her mind then she will retain control over the length and the pace of the discussion, which must allow sufficient time for the interviewer to consider ideas and opinion. Is the objective, for example, to discover whether the person has the requisite qualities for the job? Is it to find out why an employee keeps on making the same mistake? Is it to encourage someone to try to work out their own answers to a problem? Whatever the objective, the interviewer has to retain control.

Listen and observe

Let the interviewee do the talking. The interviewer's role is to encourage the discussion to develop, not to rush to an early judgement. Prompting by word or gesture, and watching for key signals (whether verbal or non-verbal), all encourage the interviewee to express thoughts and views on the subject under discussion.

The interviewer must look out for significant hesitations which may express uncertainty or perhaps difficulty in finding the right word; or even an attempt to gloss over an area of ignorance, or to avoid a topic. If necessary take notes but make it obvious that you are doing so as an aid to memory and not in a semi-furtive fashion. Nothing throws a person out of stride more than an interviewer who murmurs 'I see' in a mysterious voice, and then seems to tick off some item on an unrevealed list.

Listening while someone is talking is an essential art, particularly if you can hear what is sometimes called 'the music behind the words'. Feelings are often expressed in this unconscious way and, again, can be helpful in determining the attitudes which lie behind the spoken word. 'Oh yes I'm very keen on that kind of work' may be what is said; but the tone of voice and the dull look in the eyes can indicate the real feeling. A skilled interviewer is quick to note such apparent discrepancies, which can subsequently be discussed if considered important.

Questioning

The interviewer helps the interviewee and herself by posing questions which allow ideas to flow. An open-ended question (one which starts with 'where', 'when', 'what', 'how', or 'why' such as 'What are your views about the various filing systems used in practice today?') that reveals the person's experience will be more productive than the question 'Don't you think lateral filing is better than vertical?' – to which the answer might be an unrevealing 'Yes'. The aim of the interview should be to provide the interviewee with opportunities to give of their best. To talk about what one knows, and what one considers important will be of more use to the interviewer than a list of straightforward yes or no type questions. Whilst the interviewer will be interested to follow up what seem to be weak spots, it is through encouraging discussion based on a person's strengths that the interview will be most satisfactory. In this way, a mutual confidence is created.

At the conclusion of the discussion both people should be able to answer the question 'What have *I* gained from this experience?', even if the immediate result – failure to get the job, for instance – may appear negative.

Summarizing

Part of the way in which the practice manager can retain control of the interview is to intersperse brief summaries of what, so far, has been said, e.g. 'Although this is the second occasion when Dr X has complained that you failed to let him have the patient's notes in advance, you maintain that you thought they were in his room because you couldn't locate them in the files. How can we avoid this confusion in future?' Incidentially, this is another use of the open-ended question, which offers the interviewee a chance to think and to propose solutions.

Provided that it does not sharply interrupt the flow at a crucial point, a summary from time to time can help both people to agree that what has been said has been understood. Again, this helps to strengthen the necessary rapport.

Concluding

At the end of the interview both parties should be clear about, and agree on what has been said, what will be done next, and by whom. This applies even if no firm conclusion is reached, other than an agreement to re-convene after an interval for further thought. In the case of a job interview it may be helpful to remember that 'all selection is also rejection', and that the interviewer will have formed in the other person's mind impressions which will be important, as they will be linked to views about the practice as a whole. Remember that an interviewee will see you, as the manager, and as someone who represents the practice. When the interview terminates, what impression would *you* like the other person to take away?

The setting of the interview

Earlier in the chapter reference was made to the value of putting people at ease as a means of ensuring good communication. The practice manager is responsible for thinking ahead – for planning. Therefore, the time and place of the interview needs to have just as much consideration as the holiday or work rotas which she enters on the wall chart.

The physical location in which two people can talk is important. Is the interview best carried out in the more formal atmosphere of an office (probably so if you wish to have a brief discussion with a normally loquacious and persuasive sales representative)? Maybe you will choose the office to interview an applicant, but come out from behind the barrier of the desk and sit yourself and the other person in comfortable chairs. Or you may prefer a relaxed, less formal occasion over coffee in the common room, provided that your colleagues do not intend to use it at the same time.

There is no obvious right answer to the question of where an interview should best be held. Within what is practical and possible in the circumstances of each practice, the answer must depend on what the objective is. But it is a manager's responsibility to give thought to the occasion, and therefore to the setting. A skilful manager would not hold a discussion with a distressed secretary in the middle of a busy corridor or in full view of patients in reception. The practice manager in Chapter 1 became aware that a secretary seemed not too happy, but experience indicated that an immediate talk would not help. Instead she proposed a chat, later, over lunch when it was more likely that any tension would be reduced.

Social skills relate to the behaviour of people, but always against a background which comprises other aspects of the practice business. The technical and administrative demands of the work have to be taken into account, as they too reflect the policies of the practice. It is little use for a practice to declare that it favours open discussion amongst staff, that it wishes informality to be an important keynote, and that patients are to be encouraged to discuss problems face-to-face, if in reality the cramped conditions, the inadequate furniture, and the poor sound-proofing seem to indicate precisely the opposite. The manager's social skills will only be as effective as the physical and psychological setting in which they are able to develop.

Interviewing is not only about selection for jobs. Any communication between two people is in effect an interview. To teach, to counsel are other purposes which may be carried out in the form of an interview. The points previously listed for guidance can apply, with differing emphasis depending upon the objective. The same skills are brought into play.

Teaching and learning

In Chapter 1 we saw how a manager may take on the role of an informal teacher. What kind of teaching skills are needed?

A practice manager who is, say, an expert in PAYE may have to show a colleague what income tax must be deducted from the recently engaged clerk who happens also to be a single parent. If the objective is to ensure that the staff member understands the policy and the procedure so as to be able to do the job herself next time, then the manager will take pains to achieve this. She will explain step by step, pausing to summarize and to check that the learner has grasped what has been said, and giving her a chance to do some trial runs (errors being best made in rehearsal than in the live performance). She will be asked to fulfil other teaching functions, but not necessarily as an expert in a specific subject. Some questions about the running of a practice, or about dilemmas in which individuals find themselves do not have clear-cut answers. Yet the manager can be expected to act as a teacher in helping others to work out answers for themselves. She will want to avoid making hasty assumptions about the one 'right' answer, but rather help the enquirer to clarify possible alternative solutions before choosing the one that best fits the circumstances.

In this way, people learn to approach new problems by trying to sort out what are the pros and cons of the various solutions, and to use the teacher not as the expert with the only answer, but as a sympathetic listener who will coach the individual to explore alternatives before making a choice. People do not have to rely only on the authority of the manager: they can be helped to use their own ideas, too, A manager, for example, may wish to improve the method by which repeat prescriptions are handled. Instead of telling a member of staff 'Go and do this', she could say 'look, this is what we do now; it doesn't seem to work too well. Have a look at the system and see if you can come up with some other suggestions'. This approach also takes the pressure off the manager, and releases her from the burden of too much detail. In this way she becomes free to devote more time, not just to resolving crises, but also to her co-ordinating and planning function. Teaching others how to learn is a management skill which leads to more effective management, is discussed further in Chapter 4.

Counselling skills

A sensitive manager will be aware when a colleague or a patient wants advice or guidance, and as part of her management responsibilities she will want to intervene. She may decide to do so out of mainly humanitarian considerations (e.g. when it is obvious that an individual is troubled); out of the need to find a better way to run the practice administration (e.g. when one of the clinics keeps running overtime and the waiting patients are more and more frustrated); or out of despair (e.g. that a member of staff continues to make the same error).

Opportunities to counsel present themselves frequently, although at first they may not be recognized as such. When things are going wrong a manager's first move, naturally, is to put them right. She may, however, ask herself whether her responsibility extends beyond the immediate remedy. Can she, by offering to help in a counselling role, ensure the more deep-seated reasons have also been examined, so that an individual can take further action for herself. In which case she may wish to encourage the individual to talk, knowing that counselling is not 'telling off', even if this kind of help may follow a rebuke.

The opportunity may also arise when a person asks to have a chat, hoping to clarify confusion, or simply to test out another point of view. The manager's skill is not to jump in with a quick response – 'If I were you, of course, I wouldn't do that'. The essence of counselling is that the person doing the listening acts as a kind of sounding board, prompting the other to describe how the particular problem is seen and felt; not to provide a ready answer, but to help the enquirer to find an answer. The counsellor acts as a teacher, but not as a dogmatic expert; more as a sympathetic listener encouraging the person seeking advice to explore possible solutions. The skill of counselling involves:

(1) creating the best atmosphere to allow the individual to be forthcoming;
(2) listening and watching for the signs which betray feelings (often pointers to unspoken thoughts);
(3) helping the individual to accept what is possible for *them* to do (not what the enquirer would do in the other's shoes);
(4) leaving the other with a feeling that the conclusion is an acceptable one, and has not been reached as a result of being told what to do.

From these examples of how a manager's skills are exercised with people as individuals it is clear that being alert to one's surroundings and to what people say and feel is important. The same can be said for a manager who wishes to create a good understanding and a feeling of empathy when dealing with groups, as shown in Chapter 3.

Further reading

For a more detailed survey of the topics discussed here, the reader is referred to *Skills with people,* a guide for managers by Elizabeth Sidney, Margaret Brown, and Michael Argyle, published by Hutchinson, London, 1973.

3 Communication

Communication has been a major topic of the previous chapters. In this chapter we will first consider some principles and procedures involving the practice manager, and then discuss communication in groups more generally.

WHY COMMUNICATE?

As practices get larger, and teams form, more account has to be taken of the practice as an organization, with the practice manager occupying a key position. In the first chapter she was seen as a co-ordinator, a diplomat, and mediator, concerned with people for half her time. Rules and procedures, information, and external agencies took up half of the remainder. All these parts of her role depend heavily on her skill as a communicator.

So what is communication? The dictionary definition stresses the imparting of knowledge or information. But it also includes the exchange of ideas, and this gives us a clue. Communication is a two-way process. It involves listening and receiving, as well as imparting information and feelings. It is a dynamic process, with many subtle nuances – not just an exchange of sounds or letters. Even listening is an active process, involving eye contact, and making encouraging gestures and sounds.

There are many levels of communication – the exchange of glances, the conversation, the lecture, telephone calls, letters, group meetings – all needing their own special techniques and skills. The practice manager must be good at all kinds of communication if she is to fulfil her liaison role. Northcote Parkinson (famous for his law) described people in organizations who blocked all flow of information and initiatives, and labelled them 'abominable no-men'. As practice managers they would be a total disaster. The job needs an 'admirable yes-person' – not one who just agrees with everything, but who allows and facilitates communication.

One often hears that good communication is essential, but how is it achieved? There is no easy answer for the practice manager. Much depends on her personality, and her ability to overcome barriers to communication. Can she communicate freely with busy, individualistic doctors – some who may wish to withdraw from contact, and some who may adopt a 'boss' role and just give orders? Equally can she have an easy relationship with subordinates, or with members of different professions such as health visitors? She may see doctors as powerful figures – yet her own skill and knowledge is a source of power on which they rely. If she is sensitive to this status barrier to communication, it will make her more approachable to her juniors who might otherwise be very much in awe of her. This sensitivity will allow communication to flow, so that people working together will learn about each other and each other's jobs. They will thus build up an awareness of belonging, of common identity, on which the strength of the organization depends. This must not lead to the exclusion of people outside the organization. The practice manager must communicate with many people outside the organization, and must look for links which can be strengthened. If people on the outside can see the organization as friendly, helpful, and consistent, then co-operation will be easier. But in order to achieve consistency, different members of the organization must give the same message, and this reinforces the need for good internal communication.

Let us assume that the practice manager has the ideal outgoing, friendly but firm, smiling nature. How can she be helped in her supremely challenging task?

TECHNIQUES OF COMMUNICATION IN THE PRACTICE

Aids to written communication

In Chapter 1 the value of a notepad and a diary was emphasized. Another essential tool is a good-sized board or pin-board. On this the practice manager can display doctors' consulting sessions, outside commitments, clinic times, staff rotas, and so on. A 'white-board' of hard plastic is useful for lists of patients in hospital, and important reminders. Colour coding for different types of message or urgency is valuable.

A wall-mounted year-planner is essential to display staff holidays, public holidays, or red-letter days of various kinds. A visit to other practices or businesses, or to office-equipment showrooms will provide fresh ideas.

Written messages

Messages are the life-blood of general practice. How can the practice manager design a fail-safe system, so that urgent messages are acted upon appropriately, and none get lost?

The daybook

Many practices use a day book in which all messages are recorded. Columns are included for:

    time of message;
    who message is from (e.g. name of patient);
    whom message is for (e.g. doctor or nurse);
    text of message;
    initials of person taking and passing on message;
    tick when message passed.

This method can work very well if all staff co-operate. The doctors must check the day book before they leave on their round, and when calling in later. The district nurses and health visitors must do likewise. A member of staff must be responsible for checking that all messages have been passed (or carried forward to next day) before the surgery closes for the night. An advantage is the permanent record, which may be valuable if anything goes wrong and there is an enquiry or complaint.

Memoranda

Many practices use scraps of paper or memoranda for passing messages. These may be clipped to notes, and put in action trays. Alternatively they may be transcribed into the day book. It is helpful to have a standardized and agreed procedure, that everyone understands. Colour coding is an advantage, with a different colour for each doctor. The practice manager's memo-pad can be a particularly lurid colour! It is unlikely that a rational system will result if practices rely on drug firms to supply all the message pads. Memo-pads can be bought, or cheap paper in a variety of colours may be bought for home manu-facture of memo-pads.

For formal messages, e.g. telephone messages or memoranda from the practice manager, it is helpful to have a typed or duplicated proforma, setting out the headings of information needed. If practices are unwilling to devise and make their own message pads, they can be bought from stationers. An example of a practice manager's memorandum is shown in Fig. 3.1.

When more than one copy of a message is needed, it may be helpful to have pads of NCR (no carbon required) paper. They can be made up in different coloured paper as a reminder of the destination of the copy. Practice headed notepaper can similarly be printed with an attached NCR sheet, so that a copy of the doctor's letter is always available, whether typed or hand-written.

Where messages are placed is an important part of the procedure. Each doctor and nurse may have a labelled action tray, or a large colour-coded bulldog clip with their name clearly marked. A red-inked rubber stamp marked 'urgent' may be valuable if not used too freely. Once again it falls to the practice manager to ensure that the system runs smoothly, and messages do not get overlaid by notes or advertising matter.

The doctor's desk

This brings us to a topic where the practice manager must tread delicately. Is the doctor's desk so cluttered that notes, messages, prescription pads, and letters all get jumbled up and lost? Is the desk so loaded with trivial gifts and gimmicks that its efficiency as a work-bench is impaired? With new partners, the practice manager must use a firm hand, and never allow chaos to develop. With the older partners, tact is needed, and a diplomatic moment chosen to clear the desk, and produce a nice new blotter, with perhaps a comic message on it to forestall impending wrath. Once the point has been made and agreement

```
┌─────────────────────────────────────────────────────────────┐
│                  NEWTOWN MEDICAL GROUP                       │
│                                                             │
│   TO:      Doctors, all members of staff, HVs, Sisters      │
│                                                             │
│   FROM:    Jan Brown                                        │
│                                                             │
│   DATE:    5th June                                         │
│                                                             │
│   TIME:                                                     │
├─────────────────────────────────────────────────────────────┤
│                                                             │
│   MESSAGE:  The trainee general practitioner for the year   │
│   commencing 1st August has been appointed.                 │
│                                                             │
│              Dr Joe Smith, MB.ChB.                          │
│              24 Golden Road,                                │
│              Newtown.                                       │
│                                                             │
│   Will start work on Monday 1st August but will be visiting │
│   the practice informally on 26 June and 10 July to meet    │
│   you all. Please note that Dr Smith's home telephone       │
│   number will be:              and that all telephone       │
│   lists will require to be updated.                         │
│                                                             │
│              Thank you.                                     │
│                                                             │
│                                                             │
│                              Initials:                      │
│                                J.B.                         │
└─────────────────────────────────────────────────────────────┘
```

Fig. 3.1. Example of a practice memorandum.

reached, the practice manager can ensure that staff follow a routine of desk-tidying, so that the desk is no longer used as a giant pending-tray, or a repository for distracting and unwanted advertising matter. Just as background noise makes it difficult to hear a spoken message, so irrelevant clutter detracts from the clarity of written messages.

Telephone messages

Written messages are the least personal, so can communicate less meaning and information. A telephone call carries many more words, as well as the inflexions of voice, hesitations, giggles, or anger which all help to breathe life into the message – however crackly the line. In spite of these advantages, there is the disadvantage of the intrusiveness of the telephone. The response which the caller gets may well be coloured by what was going on before the telephone rang. Is the receptionist trying to do ten things at once in a noisy office, with a bad line, and a caller who is not familiar with the telephone? Has the doctor been interrupted in the middle of a tense consultation with a distressed or angry patient? Many consultations are ruined by this sort of intrusion, which must be avoided by carefully planned and agreed procedures.

Patients value the opportunity to talk to their doctor, and many surgery visits can be saved by easy telephone access. It is reassuring for patients to ring up to report progress or just for information. If the policy is that consultations are not interrupted for non-urgent calls, then the patient must either be given a time to ring back (not always easy from a call box subject to queues), or, if on the telephone, suggest that the doctor rings back after surgery. Some requests for information or advice can be met by the practice nurse, who may be easier to interrupt. Other ways round the difficulty are for the doctor's telephone instrument to have a visual signal rather than a bell for the waiting call, or for the doctor to have a signal to the telephonist that he does not want to be inter-rupted during a particular consultation. She can then ask the patient to ring later.

Requests for home visits

When a patient requests a visit, some practices always put the call through to a doctor, so that the message is first-hand rather than second-hand, and he can better assess the urgency. Home visits are considered further in Chapter 8.

The practice manager and the telephone

If she is not careful, the practice manager may become 'telephone-happy', ringing people when they are busy, or when a letter would suffice. Once again, the intrusiveness of the telephone can be a disadvantage, when ringing someone whom one wishes to influence or ask a favour. Sometimes people's first reaction is to say no, but on second thoughts they are more accepting. In those circumstances it is far better to type a clearly-composed letter, so giving the recipient time to think, and the opportunity to ring back at their convenience. When telephoning is necessary, it may pay to test the atmosphere by a question such as 'This is Jan Brown. Is it a good moment to ask a favour (for advice etc.) – it will take three minutes – or should I call later?'.

The practice manager must always think before she telephones and must keep calls as short as possible. This saves two people's time, and one person's telephone bill. It also clears the line for use by someone who may have an urgent message to pass. Inconsequential telephone chat is one of several time-wasting devices which people use (even doctors!) when they are under stress, or feeling tired.

The choice of telephone instruments is considered in Chapter 15. When someone rings up, the recipient may have to phone someone else (e.g. for a laboratory result). It is helpful if the telephone has a 'hold' facility to make this easier.

Face-to-face communication

The practice manager has to be accessible at all times to a wide range of people. This may be one of the most difficult parts of her job to accept. She may plan her day one way, but things happen unexpectedly, so her plans are ruined. To be interrupted when doing statistical tables, to listen to a receptionist who is worried about a sick elderly relative and is requesting leave of absence, may be frustrating. But an immediate decision, and human understanding is needed, which is all part of the job. The practice manager must not allow herself to become isolated behind her office desk. How easy a trap this is to fall into, when the whole day can be absorbed by paper work and telephone calls.

Face-to-face contact is more threatening, more rewarding, but above all, more effective as a way of communication. A sensitive practice manager will be looking for all the non-verbal cues or 'body language' which are part and parcel of everyday life, and which may give away the true meaning which the words spoken may not. In addition the practice manager's interest and sincerity will be clear as daylight to the other person. Her welcoming smile may be infectious!

A good practice manager will be well-endowed with these interpersonal skills, but many of us upset people by our manners or mannerisms without being aware of it. Some 'role play' in front of a video camera may be informative and a good educational method.

It is a refreshing exercise for the practice manager to spend a session at the reception counter, to keep up her social skills with patients, and to remind herself of their problems. It is an opportunity to work more closely with the reception staff, provided that they accept her as sharing the load rather than as checking up on them.

To summarize, a checklist of essential factors in one-to-one communication follows:

(1) sensitivity and awareness;
(2) ability to see things from the other person's viewpoint;
(3) regular face-to-face meeting with all staff;
(4) accessibility to all who wish to speak face-to-face and in private;
(5) listening and consulting rather than dictating;
(6) efficient systems for everyday communication, which all understand and use.

COMMUNICATION WITH HOSPITALS AND CONSULTANTS

Second to communicating with patients come the many pathways for communication with hospitals. Again the two-way nature of communication must be stressed. Hospitals cannot expect to be used efficiently if they do not take trouble to inform practices and the public about the services provided, and ways of gaining access. Apart from some accidents, nearly all the input to hospitals is referred from general practice – and very little is understood about the referral process. Some doctors refer five times as many patients to hospital as others, and we do not know the reason for this discrepancy.

Doctors sometimes complain about the poor quality of information they get from hospitals in the form of discharge summaries and letters from out-patients departments. Hospital doctors complain equally about the information they receive. Can the practice manager help to improve this communication process?

She can first ensure that all doctors have up-to-date and easily accessible information about hospital clinics, names of new consultants, telephone numbers, etc., so that referral to a named consultant is the rule. She can also discover, by discreet enquiry, which ones have short or long waiting lists for out-patients or admission, and which undertake day surgery. If this information is not easily forthcoming, she must pester the hospital administrator till she gets it – or even pay a visit, to see what the form is.

Requests for out-patient appointments should follow the procedures advised by the hospital, in order to make their job as easy as possible.

Letters accompanying patients to hospital, whether out-patient or in-patient, should be typed, and contain full information from the notes, such as past illnesses, social problems, current medication, allergies, and so on, where relevant. If the practice has typed summaries, the secretary can include a photocopy, so the doctor's letter need be concerned only with the immediate problem.

There is no better way of communicating with the hospital than for the doctor, health visitor, or district nurse to visit patients in hospital. The practice manager can facilitate this process by displaying an up-to-date list of all patients in hospital, including the name or number of the ward. A visit to the Admissions Office is also time well spent.

As hospitals, and practices get larger, there is a risk of losing the personal touch. One way of maintaining this is for the practice to hold a party every so often to which all the consultants who are commonly referred to (and their spouses) are invited. A summer party out of doors is ideal, but the important aim is to give the consultants a view of the practice and meet the staff, so that they too have a picture of the other end of the referral chain. They appreciate the gesture, and the improvement in communication and mutual esteem more than justifies the cost.

CONFIDENTIALITY

Communication has been discussed in terms of giving and receiving information. In her key role as the liaison person in the practice, the practice manager will find that she is involved directly or indirectly with highly confidential issues. The serious illness of a colleague, financial secrets of the practice, domestic problems of doctors and staff; all tax her powers of discretion. Confidentiality can be an enforced rule, but the examples of the doctors and of the practice manager set the tone. If they are in the habit of gossiping over coffee, then they should not be surprised if confidential information leaks out. The image of the practice is seriously harmed by a single leak of information. The consequences for staff of any breaches of confidentiality, are discussed in Chapter 2.

A good working rule is that confidential information should be given only to those who need to know and should not be bandied about light-heartedly in the hearing of people who might not be able to keep a secret. Clear procedures must be drawn up about what can and cannot be told to enquirers. For example, interested relatives may try to discover the result of a pregnancy test, and innocent enquirers after the address of patients who have moved may be debt-collectors. Information about employees should not be given to employers without specific consent. Confidentiality is considered further in Chapter 11 (p. 155).

COMPLAINTS

In the best-run practices things will sometimes go wrong. The patient, or the receptionist, or the doctor may be having a bad day. Or patients may come with unrealistic expectations which are difficult to meet, and tempers get frayed. With the diplomacy, tact, and social skills with which we have endowed the practice manager, squalls should soon subside. However, every now and again the patient or relative may complain. All complaints must be taken seriously and sypathetically however unjustified they seem, or the aggrieved party will take them elsewhere, with a consequent escalation of wasted time and trouble. This is an important part of the manager's monitoring role.

The practice manager must ensure that all staff know the patients' rights – to be seen by a doctor, to complain, and so on. These are spelled out in *Patients rights* (NCC 1982). † The complainant should be offered the opportunity to talk to the practice manager, and to their doctor – who in any case should be informed. The practice manager should unobtrusively record the patient's name and address, the date and time of the complaint and of the incident which gave rise to it, the nature of the complaint, names of witnesses, and what action has been taken.

Prevention of complaints is better than cure. There is evidence that a patient participation group (see Chapter 6) may be a good way of preventing complaints, or defusing them at an early stage. Most complainants do not want to punish the doctor or staff – they just want to prevent their unpleasant experience being repeated, so listening with humility is more effective than a defensive stance. Complaints from relatives are not uncommon after someone has died. This may be part of the grief and guilt process and must be handled with sympathy, however upsetting it might be for the staff concerned.

† Published by the National Consumer Council, and available from Community Health Councils. Republished by HMSO (1983).

WIDER COMMUNICATION

Most of the communication described so far has been between two people. It has been stressed that face-to-face communication is in general more effective than telephoning, which in turn may be more effective than writing.

The same applies when communicating with a group of people. Much of the practice manager's time will be spent with groups – whether in formal meetings or informally. But there are occasions when the practice manager must communicate in writing with many people. These are usually in the form of notices (already mentioned), procedures, and newsletters. Handouts for patients are considered in Chapter 11.

Procedures

Written procedures are essential for good management, nursing, and medicine in order to ensure clarity of thought and action. They may vary from a check-list, to a list of instructions, or a detailed algorithm or decision tree (see p. 122). the advantage of an algorithm is that it is more likely to cover all eventualities. Even if the final procedure is in the form of a list, the process of constructing an algorithm will have made sure that all loopholes for doubt have been closed. Examples of procedures will be found in Appendices A–D.

Newsletter

Even small practices can benefit from a newsletter. This can help to confirm the practice identity, and make it easier for part-time staff to feel that they belong. It can help a new staff member, coming as a stranger into a closely-knit community with unknown rules and norms of behaviour, to get the feel of the way things are. It can convey these points best if it is light-hearted in tone, but still includes vital information for all who might be interested. A newsletter can cover such topics as:

information about changes in the practice, or the community served;
details of new members of staff, with a message of welcome;
details of staff off sick, leaving, retiring, etc., with goodwill messages;
changes in time-tabling in practice, or hospital clinics and procedures;
statistical information about practice (e.g. heavy workload in previous month with congratulations to staff for coping);
any thanks from patients;
information about practice aims, research, etc.;
some light relief – cartoons, letters, competition, crossword, spoof agony column, etc.;
something to raise and maintain morale.

Not only will a newsletter help morale and communication in the organization, it will generate response from the staff, so the practice manager will be able to gain more insight into the way things are running – to help her keep her finger on the pulse of all the members of the practice, and communicate this back to them. Another example of the two-way process.

The manager and groups

There are times when we do not wish to be bothered about other people's views or feelings but simply want to set about the job in hand. To have to take other people into account seems a constraint when we can more readily act on our own initiative. The point about working in groups is not whether it is good or bad, but whether the task will be completed better by one person working alone or by a number together. The answer is rarely a stark choice between the two alternatives, but a combination of the two.

When a group of people have work to do together there is nearly always a point at which division of responsibility means assigning individual tasks. The skill of managing a group is making sure that the various parts make a complete whole when they are put together. This cannot be done unless all those involved have the same grasp of what the purpose is and what is required of each contributor. Individual skills have to relate to each other; groups rely on individuals for a collective result. A practice manager is at the same time an individual with specific authority and responsibilities while being a member of a group which can share these responsibilities. This balance between the individual and the group requires social skills.

A common fallacy is that membership of a group means involvement in a kind of extended series of committee meetings. A committee, clearly, is one form of group where a manager's skills are brought into play in order that the best use can be made of talents and knowledge. A truly effective group, however, is frequently one which survives with a minimum of formal meetings because it has taken time and trouble at the outset to understand *what* it intends to achieve, *how* it will do this, including what means of communication it will use in order to guarantee cohesion. From time to time its members come together to review progress.

Types of group

Other forms of group which a practice manager is likely to encounter will include *task groups*, which are set up to deal with a specific objective and which probably have a quite small membership; large *organizations,* such as a health centre or hospital where a number of disciplines are represented and where skills of co-ordination are essential; *functional groups*, such as the doctors in a partnership, the nurses, the receptionists, etc., each of which has its own professional expertise and ways of working, but which has to work in conjunction with the other groups to achieve the aim of providing good health care.

A manager may consider *social groups* to have an important influence on the work of a practice, even though the purpose of the group may not directly bear upon the work. Some practices regularly arrange out-of-hours leisure activities such as swimming, theatre visits, or, in one particular practice even an occasional day trip to France! This kind of group can help to cement work relationships and provides different members of the staff with an opportunity to exercise their own organizing skills. The manager may recognize latent talents which she may be happy to call on when delegation of work becomes necessary. It could be said that there are social skills in being a member of any group, whether or not one has a management role.

Whatever the group's purpose the manager will want to consider the following questions:

(1) what is the group hoping to achieve?;
(2) does it have sufficient resources within itself (e.g. knowledge, skills, experience)?;
(3) who will take any action which is agreed, and when?;
(4) what are likely to be the effects beyond the group of any decisions taken?;
(5) how will it check results?

These apply whether a group is a formally constituted meeting with a chairman, or whether it is an informal gathering of the doctors and the manager over morning coffee to discuss, for example, the need for extra staff. In any group differing points of view will have to be taken into account as work proceeds, whether this is discussion or action.

The practice manager, as noted earlier, has a responsibility for conducting meetings and for providing liaison between the staff and the doctors. Practice managers themselves recognize their roles as mediators and co-ordinators. They must be able to set the scene, so that people from different backgrounds and with different skills can work effectively together. The practice manager does not have a merely procedural function, to provide the pens and paper, as it were, for the various meetings. Because of her central role in the practice she is able to give encouragement, to raise questions, to monitor performance and, above all, to know what is required because she is attuned to the reactions and the feelings of people.

This does not mean that she has to adopt a cool, neutral stance on all matters as if she were not emotionally involved herself in the work of the practice and its inevitable effects upon the way people feel. She is aware of what is happening throughout the group as a whole, as well as within the sub-groups, be they her own administrative staff or the friendship-groups, those informal alliances which cut across work boundaries. Her awareness enables her to spot the source of potential trouble; she notes changes in her colleagues' manners, perhaps in discussions held at practice meetings. She will be able to raise questions on the group's behalf in order to clarify what may be key but underlying issues. She can, therefore, help the group to recognize the choices open to it, for example, a regular practice meeting to which everyone is invited; a small management team to represent the different sub-groups in order to deal with week-to-week business; occasional discussions between the nurses and one of the doctors, and so on. The type of group and the membership of it depend on the purpose.

Setting up meetings

The nature of general practice, with its urgent tempo and constant interruptions, makes the setting up of meetings particularly difficult. The practice manager must therefore take extra care that meetings are well prepared, and efficiently conducted with the least possible waste of time.

The John Cleese training film *Meetings bloody meetings*† gives a cruelly clear picture of what can go wrong with meetings that are not properly managed. Five steps on how to run a meeting are described in the film:

Planning ahead. What is the meeting trying to achieve? Think through the objectives.

Pre-notification. Tell those who are coming to the meeting what is to be discussed and why – concisely and in good time.

Preparation. The agenda must be in proper sequence, when one decision affects another. Time must be allocated and rationed according to the importance of the subject.

Processing. Discussion of each item needs some structure, so that people do not stray from the point, repeat themselves, or indulge in private conversation. The chairman must understand group behaviour and ensure the conflict is creative rather than destructive.

Putting it on record. A clear summary of events, decisions made; and action to be taken and by whom.

Many practices meet over lunch, as the only time they can spare. The manager must ensure that all potential attenders know the date and time of the meeting, and what is to be discussed. Any information or papers should be sent with the agenda. Items for discussion should be requested in advance, though 'any other business' is a useful slot if time allows. It should not be discussed before its place on the agenda (except in extreme urgency) or chaos will ensue. Members should be reminded of the meeting a few days ahead if it is important.

Business meetings run better if they are properly set up, with tables for papers, and seats in a circle or square, so all can see the chairman and each other. Any reference books or information should be available. The practice manager will have to consider what questions might be asked, and have the answers ready. The chairman must ensure that everyone knows how much time is allotted to each item so that the business will be completed before people start to drift away. He will need great skill to complete the business of the meeting without stifling discussion, otherwise some people will not feel committed to

† Published by Video-Arts (see Appendix F).

the decision, and so will not implement it willingly.† The practice manager must work closely with the chairman and brief him for the meeting, without giving the impression of collusion. However the practice manager may well find herself in the chair and this topic is considered next.

Being chairman

When she herself acts as chairman of a meeting the practice manager can make certain that anyone wishing to contribute an idea is not discouraged from doing so, while at the same time she must watch for domination by any one person. This is part of her *enabling* function, which is important for the development of trust and confidence in a group. An effective way to do this is not simply to go round the group asking each in turn for a view, but to encourage whoever may indicate a desire to speak to do so. She will respect the need for silence, too, and so refrain from insisting that everyone has to be involved. Her action helps to create the kind of climate in the group which is neither 'laissez-faire' – where it does not seem to matter whether one speaks or not – nor one of undue pressure. Individual differences are respected and open discussion is encouraged.

The establishment of trust takes time, especially if the group members' previous experience has taught them to hold back and remain uncommitted. Some groups find it easier, for this reason, to transact business outside formal meetings. A manager will soon become aware if serious issues which have gradually become the subject of underlying concern are avoided at these meetings, to be aired only in private. This may present her with opportunities to take on the role of a discreet mediator, whom everyone trusts because she is known to listen to the pros and cons of any argument. Whatever the purpose of a meeting, the manager has to ensure that what has been agreed is understood. She acts as a monitor for the practice.

Being chairman may come naturally to some, but most people have to learn by experience. Can they be helped by analysing the skills needed, and seeing how they can improve their performance?

One objective of the meeting is to make decisions. Not only must the decisions be as rational as possible, but they must be accepted by the group – in particular by those who have to carry out the decision. Otherwise there may be a decision on paper, but no subsequent action.

Five stages have been described for reaching decisions at meetings. They are:

(1) defining the aim;
(2) examining the information;
(3) generating alternative solutions;
(4) making the decision (using a logical sequence, if there are other connected topics on the agenda);
(5) reviewing and revising at a later stage.

---

†Further information about running meetings is available from: in Locke, Michael (1980). *How to run committees and meetings.* London. Papermac. Also from: Pemberton, M. (1982). *Guide to effective meetings.* The Industrial Society. (See end of chapter for address.)

The chairman can prepare for the meeting by ensuring that the objective is clear, the facts are known, alternative solutions have been thought through, the sequence of items has been worked out, the pros and cons have been balanced, and that arrangements for review have been considered. Further mention of decision making will be found in Chapters 7 and 16.

The chairman has a complex role. She must start the meeting by setting the scene, and ensuring that everyone knows the purpose of the meeting and the items for discussion. A balance must be kept between controlling the meeting and the agenda, and yet allowing freedom of expression and flexibility. The chairman must look for areas of agreement, and reflect and summarize progress towards a decision. All the members need to be involved in the meeting, by gesture or rapport, if not by speaking. The chairman must be free of bias, so that members' contributions can be balanced impartially. Everyone must understand the issues, so clarification may be needed. Time must not be wasted, and interest must be maintained.

As an *aide-mémoire*, the chairman can consider the following list of skills (with acknowledgement to Gordon Coote):

communicate;
control;
co-ordinate;
coax;
compare;
clarify;
concentrate.

A jocular check-list of how to disrupt group meetings might give the chair-man some insight into wrecking tactics (based on a list prepared by Shirley Otto):

arrive late: leave early;
engage in private conversations;
keep talking, even if you have nothing to say;
never volunteer for jobs, but criticize others freely;
rustle papers – or fall asleep and snore;
keep looking at your watch, tap your pen, or interrupt;
create diversions by dropping things, or passing round sandwiches, or tea;
re-open discussion about topics already decided – particularly when the meeting has finished.

MORALE

Morale in any group is based not merely on a sense of togetherness. Each individual in a group must feel valued by the group, and this sense of being valued depends on a recognition of the contribution which each person makes to the overall effectiveness of the organization. People's talents, and potential talents must be understood, as must their individual problems and sensitivities. The feeling of being an important cog in the machine is essential for morale, and the practice manager must tread carefully to keep this feeling alive in every member of staff.

Morale is more difficult to maintain where there are threats of change, and where staff turnover is rapid – itself often a consequence of low morale. It thrives on success, and is extra-sensitive to failure. It is an unstable equilibrium, so the practice manager must be particularly observant of the early signs of a lowering of morale before it becomes a landslide. This is one of the social skills already described.

Trust and confidence between people at work has to be earned by showing that approaches to the solution of problems are felt to be fair, and are not the occasion for behind-the-scenes manipulation. If the manager is to provide this kind of bridging function between different groups she will make it her business to be aware of feelings, even though she may not necessarily condone them, and will resist imposing her own feelings before people have had a chance to express themselves.

A manager who ignores or overrides her colleagues' feelings may find that groups disintegrate, that previously achieved harmony is lost, and that instead of cohesion there is a division into warring factions. Where the aims and objectives of a practice become clouded in mists of accusation and counter-accusation staff morale is low. Patients can readily detect the change in atmosphere; a tetchy receptionist might be the first outward manifestation that all is not well in the group as a whole.

Loss of morale may be due to factors other than those mentioned, resulting in a loss of group cohesion, and less-effective health care. What can a practice manager do if she detects a decline in morale?

To take a leaf out of her own book, instead of offering her counselling skills she may seek advice and guidance from a respected member of the group. She may decide to bring the whole question into the open in one of the smaller groups – probably one where she feels her views will be treated sympathetically. Nobody has to bear the burden of anxiety about morale on their own. A manager's skills also include the ability to seek appropriate help as well as giving it. As a useful guide about when to intervene she can bear in mind that if she notices a sensitive point, however unclear initially this may be, then it is most likely that others will have noticed it too. To test its reality the manager will exercise discretion in the way she intervenes. If a group member appears depressed for no clear reason, the manager will not best be served by a hasty 'you look as if you got out of bed the wrong side today'. Her skill is not only to note the signal; it is to indicate that an individual will receive a sympathetic response.

This sensitivity to group atmosphere does not mean that on every occasion when feelings are being displayed she should tactfully avoid the problem for fear of causing an upset. But the group will not respect a manager's 'bull in a china shop' tactics if these become the cause of withdrawal or unnecessary conflict. The group is then more likely to respond by closing ranks to protect a member from what may seem to be an unwarranted intrusion, particularly if this stems from a person with authority. To test one's perceptions to see if they are shared by others is an important first step in finding out whether a problem exists within the group and, if so, what can realistically be done about it.

AUTHORITY AND MANAGEMENT

Most practice managers are able to adopt different roles to suit different circumstances. In the weekly staff meetings she will probably take the chair. In the doctors' meetings she will be an adviser, making recommendations rather than decisions. At work she will have to lead, to supervise, and to encourage. Here she exercises authority based on competence and knowledge which the other staff accept. This is not the same as being authoritarian. She needs the competence to underpin her authority; she also needs the social skills to exercise leadership. The two are complementary. In acting on behalf of a group she must be flexible and prepared to learn from experience. A dogmatic approach and a closed mind will not help her progress along the road to harmony or effectiveness.

The practice manager's ideas about authority may differ from those of doctors and nurses, who have all been trained in hospital. The nurses have become used to a rigid hierarchy dating back to the early religious orders which undertook nursing. Florence Nightingale, and the more recent 'Salmon' structure have maintained this chain of authority. Doctors have more freedom of action, but in hospital are still constrained by their seniors. The relationship between doctors and nurses used to be that of the authority figure exercising clinical judgement and prescribing treatment, and the nurse meekly accepting the doctor's word. This image of the nurse as handmaiden is giving way to that of an autonomous professional who makes her own decisions in her nursing field on the advice of doctors and others. Health visitors and district nurses have probably made greater progress towards autonomy than their colleagues in hospital. General practitioners are themselves free of hierarchical constraints, and do not need to hang on to power within the organization. They have enough, and some to spare. However, old habits die hard, and may give rise to much resentment. The practice manager will have to be sensitive to these powerful forces at work in the team.

In summary we see the practice manager in her relationships with groups having similar qualities and needing similar skills to those described in earlier chapters. In particular she will need:

an ability to listen and observe;
an ability to live with uncertainty;

an ability to lead when needed;
an open mind;
a sensitivity to people's behaviour in a group;
confidence in her technical competence and social skills;
an understanding of authority which allows her to exercise or accept it;
an ability to choose the right moment to intervene;
an ability to learn from experience.

Learning and training are central issues in management, which will be considered in Chapter 4.

FURTHER READING ON COMMUNICATION

The Industrial Society publishes a set of Guides to Communication Skills, which are recommended. Available from The Industrial Society, Freepost, London SW1Y 5BR.

4 Learning and training

WHOSE RESPONSIBILITY?

Galileo is reported to have said 'You cannot teach a man anything, you can only help him to find it within himself'. As noted in Chapter 2, a practice manager needs the skills of a teacher to help her staff develop their own expertise. She can also be a wise counsellor to staff and to the partners who employ her to manage the practice.

To perform this teaching and counselling role adequately she owes it to herself to learn how to learn, and will therefore need to take opportunities to increase her own knowledge and skills. Given that all learning must come from within, the practice manager-as-teacher knows that her responsibilities are:

(1) to encourage her colleagues to acquire and to apply knowledge;
(2) to create the conditions where this can happen;
(3) to remain open and receptive herself to new ideas.

Training activities fall broadly into two categories, 'on the job' or 'off the job'. They are not mutually exclusive; the manager's role is to ensure that her staff can learn through her skill at balancing the different but complementary advantages of both kinds of training. External courses, a series of lectures, or a seminar on a particular subject must reinforce the informal but continuous learning that inevitably takes place day by day. All training must be seen as an integral part of the practice plans. Members of staff will have to be encouraged to be learning-minded.

'ON THE JOB' LEARNING

Whilst a range of techniques or teaching aids can assist the manager who wishes to stimulate learning from the experiences of the practice itself, she knows that no one method will in itself guarantee success. The use of programmed texts (often called teaching machines) may help a learner to sit quietly in a corner and try out answers to the questions posed; a video cassette, a film strip, or case studies, and even the old-style 'chalk and talk' play their part. They can profitably be used as aids to discussion, perhaps during a lunch-time meeting once a fortnight. Sources of audio-visual training aids are listed at the end of this chapter. The practice manager, whether she operated the equipment herself or delegates the task to an expert, remains responsible for ensuring that the learners, herself included, can apply what has been learnt to the real world of the practice. To learn is to receive new ideas and new information; to apply what is newly acquired and therefore unfamiliar may be to take a risk. The manager must support her learners who may feel as if they have been thrown in at the deep end. She ensures that guidance is available to them, especially in the early stages. By monitoring a learner's performance and by reviewing together each new experience in a systematic way, the manager will obtain good results because the learner will gain confidence.

The manager has to find the middle road between leaving the learner to find out the hard way and being herself over-protective. A clerk's first attempt to apply the recommendations of the 'Red Book', or a new receptionists's first experience of dealing with anxious patients, provide both manager and staff with opportunities to learn. The manager must ensure that such opportunities form part of her training plans, as the 'Red Book' cannot be left to a learner to read and absorb, cover to cover, like a novel; neither can a filmed case-study on how to receive patients be a substitute for the real thing. The manager-as-teacher will need to refer to them to reinforce good practice or to help correct errors.

In ensuring that her learner can consolidate facts she will also pay regard to that other aspect of learning – the need to understand the part feelings play in influencing the degree to which lessons are absorbed. Patients, managers, and receptionists will have their own logic, and each be convinced that their behaviour is reasonable. Emotions, however, can blur reason and the possibility of learning may be temporarily blocked. *All* learning involves both the head and the heart. A good practice manager, who will have daily experience of this herself, will encourage the learner to recognize that this is all part of learning.

When she reviews experiences with whoever is new to the particular job, the manager will want to use specific incidents to illustrate her teaching. In doing so she will want to avoid a too hasty judgement if errors have been made. Each of us will probably remember how we avoided sticking our necks out at school if punishment rather then encouragement followed our mistakes. A practice manager cannot afford to have mistakes covered up in the management of health care and so her behaviour as a teacher must create trust in her amongst her staff.

Counselling skills, as shown in Chapter 2, can play their part in assisting the learner to learn and the manager to understand what lies behind a repeated inability to apply a particular lesson. Her guidance and advice are both important and valuable to the learner, whether the occasion is one to reinforce good practice or to understand and correct errors.

A practice manager must remain sensitive to the existence of different perspectives between her colleagues and between patients. As shown in Chapter 2, sensitivity to the effects of change forms the basis for the development of management skills. This sensitivity, which includes awareness of how people react in certain situations, does not mean that a manager becomes incapable of taking necessary action.

When faced with the prospect that a learner may not be able to adapt, the manager, after gentle persuasion and attempts to encourage, must decide whether to persist or whether the learner is more suited to another kind of role. A receptionist, however well-intentioned, who insists on advising a caller to continue with aspirins for a headache graphically described over the telephone, would be demonstrating a failure to learn if she had been repeatedly warned not to give that kind of advice. Opportunities to encourage learning must be weighed against the risks which may be entailed, and in health-care mangement the luxury of learning from experience cannot always be permitted. Sometimes a manager-as-teacher may have to be clearly directive, with clear lessons about 'do's' and 'don'ts'.

Learning about people

In balancing the risks which teaching and learning must inevitably incur, all practice staff share the need to understand human behaviour – unpredictable though it may be. None the less, doctors, managers, receptionists, and patients can all help each other to learn from the reality of their experiences; indeed they have a responsibility to do so. One advantage of patient participation (see Chapter 6) is that the professionals who run the practice can learn from the patients' observations, and the latter can better appreciate the viewpoint of those who administer primary care.

If people are to learn from their experiences, sufficient time must be allowed to review and to absorb the lessons. One way to exchange ideas and feelings is to have regular, if not too frequent, discussions in small groups. This can increase the knowledge and wisdom of the practice, as well as allowing participants to use their social skills. Learning is most effective in this kind of context where the discussion topic is a live issue affecting the practice as a whole. What lessons about people might be drawn from such a discussion?

First, the content, or *substance* of the matter under discussion must be such as to enable those present to contribute. An example might be an anxious and distressed patient whose circumstances are known to the doctor, to the district nurse who has visited the home, to the social worker who has advised on rent rebates, say, and to the receptionist who may have been subjected to lengthy if confused explanations about the patient's health. There is, of course, a need to respect any patient's wish for confidentiality, but where different members of the practice in their respective roles possess information which, if shared in a professional way, can complete a picture then the practice learns, and in the long term so may the patient. The doctor may be in a position to inform his colleagues about the nature of the illness, which will enable everyone involved to respond more sensitively to the individual. All will have learnt from the sharing of knowledge and be better equipped to deal with distress.

Secondly, a group which takes such a topic as a means to learn about others may also come to learn more about itself. In addressing a specific problem people with complementary roles, such as those who comprise a health-care team, have the chance to study their own behaviour. At a fairly obvious level they can understand more about each other as people and the way they think and feel as individuals. They can also better appreciate the importance for a professional group to value the interdependence of work roles, and so they learn how to make use of each other's knowledge and skill. At a less obvious level a group, with help from its own members, can learn how to absorb influences from each other, especially by coming to recognize leadership roles which different members can take according to circumstances.

The way in which decisions are made can be another example of learning about behaviour. In certain technical matters the distinctive competence of doctor or nurse may dominate; in other cases, where no clear-cut issue is apparent, a wider-ranging, more participative approach may be desirable. In exploring its members' feelings and allowing full rein for emotional expression the group learns how tolerant it can be and what kinds of limits it places upon such tolerance for individuals.

Group discussions are vehicles for learning about leadership, and about roles which help the discussion (who summarizes, who obliges the group to pause and reflect, who points out the options for any decision, and is it necessarily always the same person?). These are just some briefly stated examples of how a practice team can learn not only from the behaviour of others (i.e. patients), but from itself.

Although the exercise of social skills is essential for all who play a part in delivering and managing health care, the receptionist represents for most patients their first contact with a practice. Yet she may be the one whose training is most frequently neglected, and therefore a separate section, towards the end of this chapter, deals with receptionists' training.

Learning and change

New habits, new methods of work, and the need for more knowledge all represent a potentially exciting challenge. They may also be felt as a threat to well-established practice; this depends on how change is perceived and how individuals see themselves affected.

A practice manager who is responsible for training others as well as herself knows that learning can be a process of discovery which can lead to the implementation of ideas, provided that the transition period, however brief, is acknowledged as having an effect upon acceptance of change. Feelings of acceptance and rejection are aroused; sometimes simultaneously in the same person. For a doctor to feel obliged to admit that a new form of treatment may prove more effective; or for a receptionist to revise, however reluctantly, beliefs about minorities, requires a change in behaviour. This is a difficult adaptation to make because it is a radical change, involving entrenched, even cherished values about what is right or wrong. Time is needed for new ideas to be absorbed. Such changes mean that an individual has to give up something fundamental. The practice manager can act as a catalyst to help this kind of learning to evolve. Where professional groupings may have been in the habit of ascribing rigid behaviour to others she may be seen as the person having no particular axe to grind.

If patients, too, are to learn how to adapt their behaviour by taking responsibility for their own health care, in conjunction with the health professionals, then old habits and beliefs will have to be discarded. Whatever their role in the health-care process, people will have to learn how to cope with feelings, their own and those of the patients; and about the merits of new as against old ways of working.

New skills will be needed; some of the almost water-tight compartments into which groups have been divided and in which they have lived and worked, will no longer be adequate. To learn how to share thoughts and feelings, to risk introducing new proposals, may present practices with problems, if the habit of being interdependent has not been learnt. Perhaps the manager is a good person to help the practice to work in closer collaboration by encouraging the development of communication skills, between individuals or between groups.

Opportunities to learn will present themselves 'on the job' probably when a particular incident, a crisis even, has to be discussed openly and frankly. The skilful manager, once feelings have been allowed expression, is in a good position to encourage her colleagues to take advantage of the incident in order to see if they can act differently henceforth.

'OFF THE JOB' LEARNING

The purpose here is not to provide readers with a comprehensive and recommended list of training courses and institutions. The relevant professional bodies, in particular AMSPAR and AHCPA, can supply details of those academic institutions with whom they have designed courses for practice managers, medical secretaries, and receptionists. Their addresses are given in Appendix F.

A further source of information is the report of a workshop held in October 1981 under the auspices of the King's Fund Centre, entitled 'Management education and primary care'. This report enables the reader to compare a number of different but complementary methods for equipping practices and health centres with the requisite knowledge and skills. The report emphasizes the value of linking theory with practice through projects which are undertaken at the place of work. Some form of 'day-release' is ideally suited, because the learner is able not only to practise what is preached but also to try out new ideas, with support at college and work. The choice of college will depend on its accessibility, the reputation of its particular teaching methods and of the tutors themselves, and on the relevance of the syllabus to the needs of the individual and the practice. But even the best courses may be only as good as the opportunity which the learner has to apply her new-found knowledge and skill. The practice manager, in her teaching role, must provide the learner with a setting conducive to trying out these lessons.

The degree to which a manager is regarded as a good teacher will in part depend on her own willingness to keep her knowledge and skills up to date. She, too, will benefit from attending courses, or discussions, held 'off the job'. A teacher needs, perhaps at least once a year, to renew the habit of learning by being herself a learner and by contributing from her experience to the learning of colleagues who are similarly engaged in the management of health care in other practices.

A design for learning and teaching

In Chapters 1 and 2 we saw what a practice manager might typically be expected to do, together with the kinds of knowledge and skills required. Her experience and the questions she may have about her role are invaluable as a starting point to encourage learning. For this reason one form of training which makes use of experience in this way can act as a model for the development of practice managers. Such a model is not a substitute for other, perhaps more familiar, direct teaching methods, but is one way for managers to explore the nature of their own roles and their function in the primary care team. In so doing the manager can practise the social skills associated with the management of people at work. This form of management training is becoming more widely used in commercial and industrial enterprises (see the list at the end of the chapter).

The principal feature is group work, in which participants have a dual task, in groups of up to 12 people, to (a) define their roles, the problems encountered, and their training needs, and (b) learn about management from the experience of having to manage their groups. Tutors are assigned to each group to assist with both tasks, although the emphasis tends to be on the skills of communicating within and between the groups. Theory and concepts about management are presented by the tutors, both in the group work and in plenary discussions.

The purpose, to quote a typical course programme, is 'to help participants to define their own needs and to assist them in finding ways of achieving the goals which they themselves have set'. Responsibility for their own learning is placed firmly on the shoulders of participants. The tutor's role is to encourage periodic reviews of what is being achieved, both in terms of the content of the discussions and the lessons about how the groups are managing themselves. Thus it is possible to see how authority is used by the group; how leadership applies to both tasks; how people communicate, verbally and non-verbally, within and between groups; how decision-making is handled; and how skills of listening and observing are used – all essential for a competent practice manager to understand.

The course ends on a practical note, with participants making plans to implement ideas back at the practice, or to arrange further training in specific subjects, the need for which they themselves have determined. †

† This method for training practice managers and senior staff was used by Oxford RHA in conjunction with the Thames Valley Faculty, RCGP and is described in the King's Fund Report 'Management education and primary care' KFC 82/6, obtainable from the King's Fund Centre, 126 Albert Street, London NW1 7NF.

TRAINING COURSES

Setting up a training course

Many practice managers have grown into their job, from previous work as a secretary or receptionist and few have had formal management training, or a management qualification. Accordingly the demand for training is very strong, both in-service training for those already in a post, and initial training for those seeking or starting work as a practice manager. Organizations such as AMSPAR and ACHPA (see Appendix F) go some way towards meeting this need, as do some NHS training institutions or departments, and colleges of further education.

If no training facilities are available in a locality there is no reason why a practice manager should not organize a course. Advice can be sought from all the organizations mentioned, and the local faculty of the Royal College of General Practitioners, and the local District or Regional Training Officer, about sponsoring such a course. It must be sponsored by a 'local education authority, local faculty of RCGP or health authority' to qualify for 70 per cent re-imbursement of fees and expenses ('Red Book', paragraph 52.9b).

A partnership is essential between those with the skills to teach, the sponsoring institution, and the people who express a need for training. The perceived needs, the expertise, and the resources must match one another if frustration is to be minimized. So what steps should be taken to set up such a training course? Ten steps are listed in Table 4.1, and are amplified in the next few pages.

Table 4.1. *Steps in organizing a training course.*

1. For whom is it intended? What needs for training in knowledge, skills, and attitudes do they perceive?
2. How many trainees can be accepted?
3. What are the objectives of the training course?
4. Agree on methods, and design course.
5. Agree staffing – tutors, lecturers, etc.
6. Allocate administrative responsibility.
7. Invite participants, indicating objectives and any pre-course work.
8. Implement course, replanning as it proceeds if necessary.
9. Evaluate course.
10. Provide methods to help apply the lessons learned on the course in practice; follow up, and plan further action.

Definition of needs

In preparing a course the organizers must be clear about the participants the course is designed to attract, and the nature of their jobs. To mix junior clerks with practice managers may not be helpful – their needs, and certainly their experiences, are likely to be different.

Is a course, for example, aimed primarily to extend the knowledge of practice managers about employment legislation and its relevance to their jobs? Or, is it aimed to improve social skills – how to handle distressed patients, provide motivation at work for the manager's subordinates, or how best to help a harassed doctor?

Whatever the training needs, clarity beforehand is essential because of implications for the design of the course, the kinds of expertise required of tutors, and the facilities to be used (video machine, flip-charts, small discussion-group rooms, etc.).

To ensure the best match between course aims and participants' expectations, the organizers are advised to seek from each participant a job profile and a description of training needs as they see them. One useful question is 'what parts of your job do you find most difficult?'.

Numbers

The size of a course is obviously important as different arrangements apply, say, to an audience of 100 people or more, or to a group of 20 where individuals may feel less like being one in an anonymous crowd. Information can be given to large numbers through a variety of methods (overhead projectors, talk, film, or a combination of these); face-to-face discussion can take place only in small groups.

Numbers relate to objectives and methods but also to numbers of staff on the course and the size of the venue itself, and, most important, to the cost. A training centre which caters for a large number of people will be less costly if used to capacity than if half-full. On the other hand the course organizers will want to strike a balance between costs and the desirability of attaining objectives. It is not much use filling a place in order to ensure revenue if in so doing the learning objectives are inhibited.

Objectives

In preparing a course, objectives have to be spelt out in advance of any invitations. It is worthwhile for the course organizers and tutors to spend time making sure these are understood and accepted, otherwise confusion is likely to arise amongst the participants. For example, while it is possible to offer both knowledge and skills training in one course, the blend of staff expertise has to be agreed in advance and staff members clear about who is best equipped to deal with specific elements in the course programme. Clarity of objectives is also essential for the subsequent review and evaluation, for participants and staff alike, when the success or otherwise of the course is to be considered.

None of this preparation means that people who are invited to attend must have exactly the same expectations. Opportunity can be taken during the course itself to check any glaring mis-match. Indeed, in determining the objectives the course organizers will need to be clear about the extent to which individual, as well as group expectations, are to be met.

Design and methods

These relate to objectives and to the training needs as expressed by participants. If there is to be opportunity for discussion and for practice then, for example, both individual and small group work has to be included in the programme. The course organizers may wish to emphasize methods and skills like counselling, interviewing, and role-playing, in contrast to lectures or visual presentation of theories and concepts. The course design must appear as an integrated pattern of activities, not merely a haphazard collection of events based solely on the availability of experts. The implication in designing a course for numbers and kinds of staff are obvious – their expertise and skills must relate to the programme as a whole, as well as to the separate elements which comprise it.

Many courses are renowned for the sheer volume of activities which they contain, but fail to take account of the value to staff and participants of un-programmed time. Participants not only learn from each other in the informal atmosphere of leisure activity, be this over drinks in the bar or walking and talking in the vitally necessary fresh air, they need the opportunity to absorb what has been presented and in the literal sense of the word to engage in re-creation. The quality of learning does not necessarily relate to quantity.

Staff

Roles of course staff, as well as numbers, have to be clear. Discussions beforehand are desirable about who does what. Are all staff members to participate in everything? (e.g. attend plenary sessions even if they may not directly take part – a valuable exercise none the less). Whether or not they attend, staff and participants must be clear about the roles to which have been assigned – X will be responsible for all plenary meetings, talks, etc; Y will ensure that periodic exchange of ideas between the members of staff takes place; Z will deal with the film and discussion or the case study.

If external speakers are to be invited as part-time course staff, engaged for a specific part of the programme, then care must be taken that any such intervention is felt to be relevant to that particular stage in the course. Course organizers are responsible for ensuring that input has a bearing on what participants require; timing is important.

Administration

Allocation of responsibility for all administrative matters is essential. A successful course is like good theatre; what goes on behind the scenes can greatly influence the result. Tutors and the administrative staff are partners.

To allow tutors or teachers to concentrate on their work it is advisable to appoint someone as course administrator. She will look after everything, from printing the programmes, sending out invitations, to agreeing domestic arrangements – catering, allocation of rooms, etc. – necessary to support the course objectives. The administrator should be present in the early stages of planning a course and be encouraged to take part in the preparatory discussions when the course is being designed.

Invitations to members

These should clearly indicate the course objectives, its methods, numbers attending, time of arrival, travel arrangements (where applicable), meal times, and also any unprogrammed or leisure time. People are entitled to know when, for example, they can expect to telephone home. The fee must be stated, and methods of reimbursement explained.

Invitations may be accompanied by a questionnaire asking participants to assist with the early stages of the course by indicating what they expect to achieve and to learn. The data collected in this way can be shared at the outset and can help participants to see the range of needs or problems that people have. Such data can be presented without attribution to individuals.

Implementation of the course

Objectives should be reiterated at the beginning, administrative arrangements confirmed, course methods explained, staff members introduced, and questions for clarification invited. This is an important element as it can help participants to feel their way into what may be, for many, a strange or unusual setting.

Evaluation

This should be carried out against the declared objectives, and should include the course as a whole as well as its separate elements. However, evaluation is an integral part of the process as the course develops, and opportunities will occur for members of staff to review experiences with both individuals and groups.

The course organizers, if they listen and learn from what happens during the course, may decide to make changes – to include or omit a particular activity. Evaluation is continuous therefore, which does not mean examining the plant every hour to see if it is still growing!

At the end of the course participants should be encouraged to make their comments, critical or not, as they feel at that time. At a later stage, say 3–6 months afterwards, a more reflective evaluation can take place through a questionnaire. Participants need time to absorb what they have learned and to assess its relevance to their own individual development and to the needs of the workplace.

Results of the evaluation should be collated, where possible discussed by the course organizers and staff, and distributed to course participants.

Application and follow-up

Before leaving the course, individuals or small groups with common interests or problems should be encouraged to think about the action which they might undertake as a result of the course.

On return to work each course member is advised to hold a de-briefing discussion with their sponsor (the senior partner, or unit manager, for example). New proposals arising from what was learnt have to be aired with colleagues. Action plans may include ideas about training 'on the job', a further course for oneself or colleagues, and certainly a report back to, say, the practice meeting about what the course had attempted. Some form of action should follow from the individual's participation in the course.

Participants with common interests may arrange their own meetings to continue to support each other and to learn from each other's experience – an important lesson from the course. Each individual should feel encouraged to try something new, however minor it may seem.

Joint training

Although practices may find it difficult for two people to be away at a course at the same time, consideration should be given to a doctor and, say, the practice manager attending together some form of joint training, as has been tried in some regions with considerable success. Doctors have financial and legal responsibilities in connection with the running of their practices. To take time to acquire fresh insights and new ideas with the person appointed to manage the practice as an entity must be worthwhile. If insufficient courses exist for this kind of joint training, then perhaps a 'do it yourself' approach would be rewarding. Learning starts where the need is felt.

General practitioners or practice managers who feel the need for further training would do well to make contact first with the training officer of the local District or Regional health authority. If this fails, an approach can be made to local colleges of further education or management training colleges. Organizations like AMSPAR and AHCPA might help, as might the King's Fund College. In addition an approach could be made to organizations operating in the industrial-training field. A list of addresses can be found at the end of this chapter.

Claiming allowances for training

Practice managers need to be conversant with the regulations about staff-training courses, so that the allowances may be claimed in full. There are two types of course which staff may attend.

1. *Courses with general practitioners* (coming under the Section 63 regulations). Staff must complete a claim on the appropriate form to cover course fee, travelling, and subsistence, if allowable.

2. *Courses arranged primarily for staff* (e.g. receptionists, secretaries, practice managers, practice nurses). Claims are made under the 'Red Book', paragraph 52-8–9. Seventy per cent of course fees, travelling, and subsistence may be claimed for courses organized by, or in association with, local education authorities, local faculties of the RCGP, or health authorities. The claims are made by the practice on the usual ANC 3 form. Practice nurses do not, at present, qualify for course fees. This is under review (1988).

In both cases the salary of direct employees while on a course attracts 70 per cent reimbursement, as does the salary of a locum, provided the limit of two employees per partner is not exceeded. If in doubt, consult the FPC or health board.

Staff employed by health authorities are equally eligible to attend these courses, but permission must be obtained from the manager concerned. The cost may need to be included in a training budget, so early application is advisable. The health authority may request the practice to pay 30 per cent of the cost at their discretion. Courses run by health authorities are often free of charge to NHS staff. Courses run by AMSPAR or ACHPA are eligible for 70 per cent reimbursement, provided they fulfil the 'Red Book' conditions.

Helpful organizations

The following organizations might help in arranging management training for GPs and/or practice managers.

Association of Medical Secretaries,
Practice Administrators, and Receptionists (AMSPAR),
Tavistock House South,
Tavistock Square,
London, WC1H 9LN.

Association of Health Centre and Practice Administrators (AHCPA),
Lord Lister Health Centre,
121 Wood Grange Road,
London, E7 0EP.

Health Services Management Centre,
University of Birmingham,
Park House,
40 Edgbaston Park Road,
Birmingham, B15 2RT.

King's Fund College,
2 Palace Court,
London, W2 4HS.

Centre for Corporate Strategy and Change,
University of Warwick,
Coventry CV4 7AL.

Royal College of General Practitioners,
14 Princes Gate,
London, SW7 1PU.

Further reading
Pritchard, P. (1988).
Training practice staff.
Horizons. **2**. 217–22 and 295–300.

TRAINING OF RECEPTIONISTS

Many practice managers will have been receptionists and some will regularly take their turn at the counter. They will know, therefore, the importance of the skills required for this 'front of house' role. A receptionist deals with people who may be under emotional stress, and who consequently expect or even demand instant attention and access to a doctor.

She records important messages accurately; answers incessant phone calls; has to exercise judgement about what is urgent; and keeps an eye open for the doctor or nurse becoming free. In between times she helps to file patients' notes and handles repeat prescriptions. A good receptionist, however, is not simply born to this kind of work with its very obvious requirements for social skills, although personality must be an important factor. Like her colleagues in the primary team the receptionist has training needs which will largely be met 'on the job'. A sensitive manager who sees teaching as one of her key responsibilities can influence strongly the development of the receptionist's own skills, together with self-confidence. She knows how important it is for the practice as a whole to be represented at the reception-desk by someone who understands behaviour and who appears helpful to the people whose health care is the concern of the team. The manager will therefore make it her business to know about training courses available for receptionists, as well as to ensure that opportunity is taken for learning from daily experience.

Courses are run by a number of colleges in association with AMSPAR, from whom details can be obtained. These are mainly day-release courses which comprise one half-day per week spread over two terms, enabling the receptionist to put into practice what she learns and to review the results with the course tutor and her manager. A typical programme includes:

   background to the job (structure of NHS; nature of the doctors' contractual
      relationship);
   administration (repeat prescriptions; records; filing systems);
   human relations and communications (receiving patients).

In the Reading area a behavioural approach to receptionists' training was made by Anderson *et al.* (1980), using transactional analysis and encounter group methods. A feature of this workshop was role-playing as a means to understand why people react in certain situations, such as the encounter between a harassed receptionist and a demanding patient. This helps role-players to experience what it feels like to take another's part. A receptionist might appreciate how the description 'awkward patient' can seem different when she herself is asked to be 'awkward'. Perspectives differ: one person's awkwardness might be another's anxiety – even though it is expressed in a bluff, aggressive manner.

To train a receptionist in, say, the techniques of response (how to remain cool, speaking firmly but gently), is only part of the answer. She really needs to understand the causes of behaviour, and one vivid method is to experience for herself the patient role.

Other methods to help the receptionist develop skills and confidence include video recordings (see pp. 272–3), film strips, or slides – all of which are useful when the theme is discussed between receptionists at a course, or at a practice meeting where different points of view can help the receptionist to understand how to play her part more effectively. Some practices have used a video camera to film the receptionist as she receives patients at the hatch. Others have used role-playing sessions where the dialogue between the patient and the receptionist is simulated. Both methods are powerful ways of illustrating the process of communication between patient and receptionist. Common to all these methods is the lesson about the influence of emotion in transactions between people. Doctor, patient, and receptionist are all, at various times, subject to pressures which will occasionally find expression in an outburst of 'blowing one's top'. The receptionist must be helped to understand that such behaviour is normal, that ways have to be found to cope with it, and that outbursts are sometimes necessary. The receptionist must learn that to seek to place blame is net very helpful. Included within the receptionist's responsibilities is that of absorbing feelings expressed by others.

Time spent by team members, including the receptionist, in discussions which give rise to mutual learning is not a luxury, but a necessary element in the team's self-development – part of its professionalism, in fact. The upkeep of knowledge and skill is just as much a practice responsibility as the upkeep of patients' notes or the fabric of the building.

The receptionist is usually the first person to be recruited by the doctors when a new surgery is about to open (Anderson and Steel 1979). Her training, whether in the use of efficient administrative systems or in the exercise of judgement about people will be an important factor in helping the development of a practice style. Training, naturally, cannot effect magic where the practice has failed to follow the appropriate staff selection procedures (see Chapter 2). In this case, training will prove an unrewarding and protracted business, resulting in frustration for the practice, the patients, and the receptionist alike. An introverted and uncommunicative person is hardly suited to receive patients sympathetically or to tolerate the inevitable whims of doctors working under pressure.

THE TRAINEE GENERAL PRACTITIONER

Vocational training has been going on for over 30 years, but it is only during the last ten years that the number of trainees has increased fivefold, to nearly 2000. Now all new entrants as principals in general practice must have undertaken three years' vocational training – two years in relevant hospital jobs, and one year in general practice. Setting up training programmes is well covered in the books quoted at the end of this section. Three facets only will be considered here:

difficulties experienced by trainees;
management support needed for the trainee and for the practice;
management training needs of the trainee.

Difficulties experienced by trainees

After many years of hard work and uncertainty, the qualified doctor does his or her pre-registration year of hospital work and then becomes fully registered. If he wishes to become a principal in general practice, there are another three years of moving about from job to job, and often moving house too. Most districts now have co-ordinated training schemes, so there is a better chance of continuous employment, but less choice of hospital jobs and practice. Some doctors prefer to vary the mix of jobs, so have to make all their own arrangements. The doctor usually knows, during the hospital jobs, which practice he will be going to, and so may make contact and become familiar with the practice and its ethos – and also with the problems being experienced by the current trainee.

The year in general practice is often thought to be less demanding than the hospital jobs, but it is a totally different environment for many doctors who have spent the previous five years or so in hospital. It may make equal demands on the doctor. Being called a 'trainee' is not helpful – it makes patients think of students. The term is best avoided in the hearing of patients by calling the trainee 'Doctor X who is working with us for a year'.

The trainee, not having a personal list of patients, will tend to see those patients who are in a hurry to see a doctor and who cannot wait to see 'their own doctor'. Trainees may also inherit patients from the previous trainee – often the high-attenders with fat folders who have been rejected by their doctor. The trainee may get less job satisfaction from seeing children with colds and incurable neurotics than to take full responsibility for people with chronic ailments. A year is not long for follow up, and usually the time available is much shorter. Yet, experience shows that it is long enough for patients to become very fond of 'the new doctor' and to be sad when he leaves. A major difficulty is the re-orientation process from hospital medicine – often dealing with crises – in which scientific medicine is practised by a group of doctors, to the more isolated and uncertain area of general practice.

Many administrative difficulties arise for the new trainee – accommodation, fixing and manning the telephone, claiming for removal and telephone expenses, filling in endless forms, getting kitted out for emergency calls. In these and other tasks the practice manager and partners need to show an example of good practice management which, one day, the trainee may follow.

What does the trainee expect of the year in practice?

Each doctor coming to the practice may have different expectations of the year. Some may be keen to take responsibility and plunge into the work; others may have research or specialist interests, or interests outside medicine altogether. Some may be involved in clinic work (e.g. family planning), some may be taking exams (e.g. DRCOG, DCH), or working for the MRCGP. Some trainees may see themselves as students doing an academic course in general practice.

The partner responsible for training will doubtless be aware of the orientation of the current trainee, and make appropriate allowances. The practice manager, too, will have to find out from the trainee what he or she expects, and try to meet these expectations as far as is practicable.

Attendance at courses, clinics, hospital sessions, and project and tutorial work will all have to be dovetailed in to the practice timetable. Once again the practice manager will find herself doing a balancing act between the needs and expectations of the trainee and those of the practice. The training partner is allowed time for tutorials and meetings; in exchange the practice gets an extra pair of hands for about half the time. If excessive service demands are made on the trainee, at the expense of the educational side of the year, it might be seen as exploitation. But short of that, the quality of the trainee's work may be lessened if he or she is used as a dogsbody and is given all the odd jobs to do, rather than a representative selection of the work that as a principal he will undertake in the future. It may be rationalized as 'giving the trainee experience', but the balance must be right.

Not only may a willing trainee get all the odd jobs, but if he or she is a good listener, may become a confidante for the staff, or even the partners, and so get more heavily involved in practice tensions than is justifiable in the circumstances.

Management support for the trainee and for the practice

As soon as the trainee is appointed the practice manager must check the date of starting, and make sure that there are no problems with the paperwork. If the trainee is still doing hospital jobs, no opportunity should be lost to encourage him or her to become involved in the practice, by attending clinical meetings, parties, or dropping in when free time is available.

On arrival the trainee must be made to feel welcome, and be introduced to all the staff. An individual plastic nameplate on the door is more welcoming than a scruffy paper label, and it establishes his or her status with patients, as does a notice in the waiting room and an individual rubber name-stamp. A consulting room for the trainee's sole use is essential, and there should be space for study and project work. Whereas a practice library may contain mostly works of reference, a training library should be well-stocked with texts suitable for the trainee, as well as books about teaching and administering the trainee year. A bibliography can be obtained from the Librarian of the Royal College of General Practitioners. The partners can delegate the purchase of books, within a budget, to the practice manager. If the trainee wants books for study he or she can approach the practice manager direct. (See Chapter 14 for more about libraries.)

The practice manager, in consultation with the partner responsible for teaching, should ensure that the trainee has as much responsibility as possible. This should be balanced against time spent on attending courses, project work, visits outside the practice, and trainee exchanges.

The practice manager must ensure that the doctor responsible for training can set time aside for tutorials, without interruption. It is helpful if teacher and trainee can have a short time together after each consulting session to review what has happened, and allocate responsibility.

Each practice and each trainee will have different needs, so a flexible approach is essential. However, a check-list may ensure that nothing is overlooked.

(1) nameplate and rubber stamp ordered;
(2) inform FPC of starting date;
(3) FPC, and NHS superannuation forms;
(4) check salary level and inform wages clerk, obtain P45 and insurance card;
(5) check telephone arrangements, and need for answering machine;
(7) arrange letter of contract for trainee;
(8) ensure that trainee is a registered medical practitioner, and a member of a defence society;
(9) help with claim forms, e.g. for car telephone, removal, or extra petrol expenses; interview and examination expenses etc. (see 'Red Book', section 38, and check with FPC);
(10) check timetable, and ensure reception staff are fully informed;
(11) arrange tutorials in practice management.

Management-training needs of trainee

Trainees take a little time to settle in and gain confidence. At first they may be overwhelmed by the strange new environment of general practice and not be too concerned with the mechanics of it. However, as the year proceeds they will come to realize that one day they will have management responsibilities and they may be asked about practice management in the RCGP examination. At an early stage the practice manager and trainee should have a session on the 'practice day' – what happens from the moment the staff arrive, the phones are switched through from night emergency, the doors open, and the headlong rush starts! This would be a 'day in the life of the organization' which the practice manager is controlling.

Much of the learning in the trainee year is opportunistic. As a problem or situation arises, it can be used for teaching. This makes a systematic coverage of a subject difficult to achieve. If the practice manager keeps a check-list of areas and topics, they can be ticked off as they are discussed and dealt with. The contents list of this book, or lists from training books may be used (see list at end of chapter). Regular tutorial session with the practice manager or partner will fill in the gaps and may have to take place at short notice – for example if the GP-teacher is called away from a tutorial session. Practical work can be arranged, such as a session as receptionist or answering the telephone, or doing the accounts. Visits to outside agencies such as the FPC, the Health Authority, etc. are an important part of training.

Joint training for the different disciplines in primary health care is an important way of building the bridges of understanding that are needed so badly. The practice manager is in a key position to arrange this. Joint visits and joint courses are one way. Lunch-time discussions using tape-slide or video teaching material are a particularly valuable way of bringing the different disciplines together. A list of libraries of audio-visual material follows the reading list.

Books useful for trainee general practitioners

Learning and teaching

Cormack, J., Marinker, M., and Morell, D. (Eds). (1981). *Teaching general practice.* Kluwer Medical, London. £18.50.

Gray, D. J. Pereira (1982). *Training for general practice.* Macdonald and Evans, Plymouth. £9.95.

Hall, M. S. (Ed) (1983). *A GP training handbook.* Blackwell, Oxford. £7.50.

RCGP. *The future general practitioner. Learning and teaching.* RCGP and BMA, 1972. £7.50.

RCGP. Bibliography on vocational training assessment.

Ronalds, C. *et al.* (Eds). (1981). Fourth national trainee conference. RCGP Occasional Paper No. 19. £2.75.

Practice organization and management

Jones, R. V. *et al.* (1985). *Running a practice,* 3rd Edn. Croom Helm. London. £10.95.

Oxford Trainee Handbook (1978). *Trainees' vade-mecum.* Blackwell Scientific, Oxford. £2.50.

Pritchard, P. M. M. (1981). *Manual of primary health care. Its nature and organization.* 2nd Edn. Oxford University Press, Oxford. £6.95.

Parr, C. W. and Williams, J. P. (Eds) (1981). *Family practitioner services and their administration.* The Institute of Health Service Managers, 75, Portland Place, London, W1N 4AN.

General Practitioner (1983/4). *The business of general practice.* (3rd edn). Prepared for General Medical Services Committee. (Has a useful section on training.)

SOURCES OF AUDIO-VISUAL MATERIAL FOR TEACHING

Graves Medical Audio-Visual Library

Holly House, 220 New London Road, Chelmsford, Essex CM2 9BJ. Tel. (0245) 83351.
An extensive series of tape-slide and video-cassette programmes suitable for general
practitioners, trainees, nurses and reception staff. Catalogue on application.

MSD Foundation

Tavistock House, Tavistock Square, London, WC1H 9JZ. Tel. 01-387-6881.
Developing a series of high-quality audio-visual programmes for general practitioners
and staff. Catalogue on application.

Video-Arts Ltd.

Dumbarton House, 68 Oxford Street, London, W1N 9LA. Tel. 01-637-7286.
John Cleese Management Training Films. Include: *Decisions, decisions. How am I
doing? Manhunt. Meetings bloody meetings. The secretary and her boss. Difficult
customers. Making your case. Do you think you can manage?* Films are expensive to
hire. The health authority training department may have a copy which can be loaned.

British Life Assurance Trust for Health Education (BLITHE)

BLAT Centre, BMA House, Tavistock Square, London, WC1H 9JP.
Clearing house for information on audio-visual aids for health and medical
education, and a large library. Now includes the BMA film library.

Health Education Authority

Hamilton House, Mabledon Place, London WC1H 9TX. Tel 01-631 0930.

Pharmaceutical companies

Many firms now have training video films which are aimed at practice staff, e.g. The
Art of the Receptionist (Professor Michael Drury), distributed by Dista Pharma-
ceuticals, Kingsclere Road, Basingstoke, Hants, RG21 2XA. Tel. (0256) 3241.

Royal College of General Practitioners

14 Princes Gate, London, SW7 1PU.
Videotape and booklet 'Management in Practice' (1987).

5 Working as a team

. . . the concept of the primary health-care team is viable and should be promoted wherever possible in the interests of improved patient care.

This was the overall view of the Joint Working Group on the Primary Health Care Team which reported recently (DHSS 1981*a*). They made 50 recommendations, of which 16 concerned communications, management of services, and organizational factors. Many of the recommendations relied for their success on good management procedures. The practice manager is essential to good team working, both as a member of certain teams, and in her central facilitating and liaison role described in Chapter 1. But before considering ways she can help teams to function better, let us ask: 'what are primary health care teams, and how do they function?'

WHAT IS A TEAM?

A team is defined as:

A group of people who make different contributions toward the achivement of a common goal.

This definition is such a broad one that most human activity can be seen as teamwork – as indeed much of it is. To clarify what we mean by teamwork in general practice, we can consider the four essential characteristics of teamwork described by Gilmore *et al.* (1974), arising from a Scottish study of primary health care.

1. The members of a team share a common purpose which binds them together and guides their actions.

2. Each member of the team has a clear understanding of his own functions and recognizes common interests.

3. The team works by pooling knowledge, skills, and resources; and all members share responsibility for outcome.

4. The effectiveness of the team is related to its capabilities to carry out its work, and its ability to manage itself as an independent group of people.

These 'essential characteristics' help us to understand the nature of teamwork. They can be used as a yardstick of good team working, if we ask ourselves:

1. Do we share a common task?

2. Are we clear about what job each of us does?

3. Do we share knowledge, skills, and responsibility?
4. Do we work as an autonomous group (i.e. without control from outside)?

The nature of primary health-care teams

The intrinsic team

Confusion has arisen in the past by thinking of 'the team' in the singular, whereas a closer look reveals that there are many different teams, pursuing many different tasks, with many different combinations of people making up the teams. Here is an example:

An elderly patient who lives with her daughter develops a stroke. The daughter telephones the general practitioner, who visits, and makes a diagnosis and a plan. He asks the district nurse to call. She makes an assessment and reports back to the doctor. They all agree that home care is advisable for the present.

This is a team consisting of the patient, the supporter (her daughter) the general practitioner, and the district nurse. The task is the management of the patient's illness at home. As the illness changes, so other team members may be involved (e.g. the health visitor or social worker) in response to different needs and tasks. So we have here the basic 'intrinsic' unit of teamworking which centres round the patient, and copes with the task in a flexible manner. (see Fig. 5.1).

As well as agreeing on the task and knowing what each team member can contribute, good procedures in communicating are needed. Here the practice manager and receptionist come into the picture: on occasions when they are part of the team, making an essential contribution.

This concept underlines the importance of the patient (and supporter) in the team. It helps to 'de-professionalize' health care – to emphasize people doing things together rather than professionals 'doing things to' patients.

Functional teams

Many other intrinsic teams exist, with different patients and groupings of staff. Clearly some co-ordination is needed. This can be achieved by periodic meetings

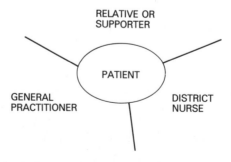

Fig. 5.1. The intrinsic team. Task: management of acute illness at home.

of, for example, the general practitioner and district nurse to review the mutual case load. Similar meetings could be held with practice nurses, health visitors, and/or social workers. These have been called 'functional' teams, because they deal with one particular function such as home nursing.

On the administrative and management side, there are three important functional teams which need to meet regularly:

(1) the partners;
(2) the practice manager and general practitioner;
(3) the reception staff and practice manger (and sometimes the general practitioner).

Some partners have such confidence in their practice manager that she attends almost all their meetings, and in this case the first two teams could be merged. This would have the advantage, mentioned in Chapter 3, of meetings being properly organized, and decisions recorded and communicated. The third team has to maintain a balance between delegating full authority to the practice manager to supervise the reception service, and loss of contact between receptionist and doctors.

Some tasks involve doctors and nurses; some involve lay staff. To suggest that there are two categories or qualities of teamwork, professional and lay, or to exclude receptionists from the primary health-care team is invidious and hurtful. The quality and dedication of teamwork is not a professional preserve.

The full team

There are occasions when all the staff in a surgery or health centre may want to meet – to co-ordinate the work of the various functional teams, or to deal with issues affecting all staff, such as the premises, holidays or parties. On these occasions the 'full team' can meet. The meetings may be crowded and out of control, so that people break up into separate groups having their own private conversations. Here the manager has to take a firm hand, by ensuring that the meetings are properly organized, and deal only with topics of common interest. If the functional team meetings are working well, then infrequent full team meetings can be successful events.

DEVELOPING TEAM WORKING

The DHSS joint working group (DHSS 1981*b*) went on to say:

successful teamwork needs more than an agreement to work together. Conscious efforts towards preparation for teamwork need to be made, both at individual team level, and during professional training.

the concept of teamwork needs to be actively promoted through continued training at all levels, particularly within a multi-disciplinary framework.

there must be a commitment to the principle of teamwork at local level by all the professional staff involved.

How can good management ensure that there is adequate preparation, active promotion, and commitment to teamwork? The problem is a big one, which has not been tackled over-all by the educational institutions, the health authorities, or by nursing management – though striking initiatives have been taken in some areas. The DHSS report, had many recommendations for health authorities and NHS management: let us consider what can be done within the practice. But first, what are the obstacles to team-working?

Obstacles to team working

Lack of commitment by general practitioners is a major obstacle. The DHSS report made the point very strongly that there were two very different viewpoints of teamworking – the doctors' and the nurses'. This may result from different training and approaches to their job, but the main difference seems to be a failure to understand each other's role, and each other's problems and expectations. There are still general practitioners who see district nurses and health visitors not as fully trained and independent professionals, but as handmaidens, ready to take orders.

If a chasm exists between general practitioners and nurses, there is likely to be an equally formidable one between the 'lay' staff and the others. A high priority is the building of bridges between these groups so that they have a closer understanding of each other's jobs. To do this requires tactful commitment to a difficult educational process. The general practitioners must take the lead, but the practice manager can play a very important part in fostering mutual understanding. Joint lunch-time meetings with an educational content (such as tape–slide material: see list at end of Chapter 4) can help to widen people's horizons and emphasize common interest's rather than divisions. In some meetings the question must be faced – 'How do we see the other's job?' Role-play can be tried, in which staff play-act the other's job when discussing a mutual problem. Another method is for staff to try to describe the other's job – the results can be hilariously wide of the mark!

Poor practice organization can be harmful to team working. The system for passing messages must be efficient, the practice manager must foster good communication, meetings must be well organized and effective, leadership must be sensitive, and people must listen. It does not help good team relationships if health visitors or social workers have to join the waiting-room queue to see the doctor, or if telephone calls are put through with bad grace or not at all.

Frequent and informal meeting helps a team to function. Daily meetings at coffee breaks, and at other times by chance, all help the sort of equal and friendly relationship for which we aim. This is, of course, much easier if team members share the same building. If this cannot be achieved, then everyone will have to make particular efforts to meet face-to-face.

Too large a team makes for greater difficulty in forging close links, as do frequent staff changes. It is as if the human organism can only manage a small number of close relationships. Small is beautiful in teamworking – hence the value of attachment of nurses to general practice, which found favour in the DHSS report.

Nurse attachment does not find universal favour with nurse managers. It makes their job more difficult, and nursing staff spend more time travelling – particularly if the doctor has a diffuse practice. Some nurse managers have eased the burden on their staff by detaching them from general practice, and running the district nursing and health visiting service on a geographical basis from a central agency. This arrangement has short-term advantages for the community nursing service, but is widely held to be harmful to the development of the primary health-care team. There would be no dilemma if general practitioners had less diffuse practices, i.e. if they only accepted patients from a defined and more compact area, preferably the same area covered by nursing staff too. This zoning of practices makes for economy in the doctors' and patients' travelling time, and may be the only way to save team working in cities. General practices which have tried it have found it beneficial.

The problem of detachment of nurses by nurse managers is a symptom of a more serious problem for teamworking, namely the divided loyalty of nurses and social workers in a team. The fourth 'essential characteristic' of teamwork described the need for the team to manage itself as an independent group of people. If the district nurses and health visitors see the employing health authority, represented by their nurse-manager, as the major focus of their loyalty, this will reduce their commitment and loyalty to the team – which is essential for its success. If we believe that teamworking makes for better patient care and greater job satisfaction, then nurse managers should do all they can to foster it. Greater clarity is needed by managers and nursing staff in defining which areas of their work are 'team' and which are 'hierarchy' †. The managers need a light touch and great skill to succeed in this balancing act. They will be helped if they have good contacts with general practice, rather than be excluded. The practice manager has a role here, in ensuring that the aims of nursing management can be made compatible with the aims of primary health care and general practice.

Confidentiality depends upon mutual trust among team members. The larger or more diffuse the team, the less opportunity will there be to develop trust, and so there will not be the sharing of information essential to teamworking. There is the opposite danger of highly confidential information being shared too freely in a team-happy group, without any mandate from patients (implicit or explicit) to disclose this information.

Newcomers to a closely-integrated team may have great difficulty in becoming part of the group and identifying with it. Particular effort needs to be made to ensure that a new staff-member settles in to the team. The practice manager's sensitivity is a key factor. Good teamworking should give better job

---

† See Chapter 16 for further discussion of these kinds of organization.

satisfaction, and a lower staff turnover, but the process does not just happen without any conscious effort.

Helping teams to work well

Several suggestions for improving teamwork by overcoming obstacles have been made. What further positive steps can be taken to facilitate teamworking? Team members often say that the most valuable feature is the 'open-ness' of a good team. This can be fostered by getting to know each other socially as well as professionally. Team parties, preferably away from the work-place, can be very rewarding.

Joint learning helps people to understand each other's jobs and aspirations. Such multi-disciplinary training is a rare event outside the practice, so practices can arrange their own, as already suggested.

Understanding how teams work, and taking time off to look at the workings of one's own team, are among the most effective ways of improving team performance. Perhaps one of the team members is a good facilitator of this process. If not, then outside help can be sought in the form of an 'organization development' consultant with experience in team development. Such an experiment was tried in eight teams in the Oxford Region, with some notable successes.

Another approach is to use team-building methods, similar to those developed in the USA, for a 'do-it-yourself' programme without outside help (Rubin *et al.* 1975). If this proves too daunting, a compromise would be to engage a consultant to get the programme started. Such a person might be seconded from the Regional Health Authority, or employed directly by the practice.

Rubin and his colleagues found that it was best to look at team processes in a particular order:

(1) Goals   – What are we here for?
                                        – What is the task?
(2) Roles   – Who does what?
(3) Procedures   – How do we go about it?
(4) Interpersonal relationships – How do we get on together?

By starting at the top of the list, teams got their working relationships going, and rarely reached the last item – interpersonal relationships – because they had already sorted themselves out. But if they started with interpersonal problems, they never reached the task!

For those with the courage to look at their own performance, a list of possible questions which team-members could ask themselves is given in Table 5.1. For delicate teams, they should be taken in small doses!

NURSING IN PRIMARY HEALTH CARE

Whatever views doctors may have about the nature of the primary health-care team, there is no doubt about the essential contribution which nurses make to

Table 5.1. *Questions about team working (drawn from several sources, in particular Argyris, G. and Beckhard, R.) From Pritchard, P. (1981).* Manual of primary health care, *2nd edn. Oxford University Press*

Aims, tasks
1. Are we all here for a common purpose?
2. What is that purpose?
3. Do we agree about the tasks we set ourselves?
4. Do we define them adequately?
5. Can they be measured, so that we know if task has been completed?

Roles
6. Are we clear about our own role in the team?
7. Are we clear about the roles of others in the team?
8. Are these roles in conflict, and if so where?
9. Are we unable to fulfil our role (e.g. due to overwork)?
10. Is our ability to carry out our role hampered by outside constraints (e.g. not being allowed to make decisions, fear of litigation, etc.)?

Procedures
11. In making decisions do we take adequate notice of:
    (a) who has the relevant information?
    (b) who has to carry out the decision?
12. Are decisions usually made:
    (a) unanimously? (b) by majority? (c) by team leader? (d) by default?
13. When a decision is made, is it carried out or forgotten?
14. Does the team follow up its decisions, question the outcome, and learn by its mistakes and successes?
15. When a conflict arises do we:
    (a) ignore it? (b) allow one person to force a decision? (c) compromise? (d) look for alternative solutions?
16. Do we let everyone have a chance to speak, or let one or two members do all the talking?
17. Does everyone feel free to challenge any statements made in the group?
18. Do we waste time, or allot it according to the priority of the task?
19. Does the team meet often enough and in the right circumstances, and is the size of the group right?
20. Do team members concentrate on the task or waste time trying to impress, or raising irrelevant issues?

Interpersonal relationships
21. Are team members sensitive to how others in the group feel about discussion?
22. Can the team tolerate failure, and give mutual support rather than blame?
23. Is team morale high? If not, why not?
24. Can any member suggest any way in which team working could be improved?

---

care of the patients in the community, be they district nurses, health visitors, nursing auxiliaries, practice nurses, or specialists such as community psychiatric nurses, geriatric liaison, paediatric, stoma care, and hospice-based nurses.

The management of the nursing profession in the community is outside the scope of this book, though the need for co-operation with nursing management has been stressed. One area, however, which general practitioners and practice staff may need to understand is the way nurses manage their work – the '*nursing process*'. This has lately become the basis of the work and teaching of nursing both in the hospital and the community. It has much in common with the ways in which other professionals manage their work.

The nursing process

This has been described as an

interactive, problem-solving, decision-making procedure for assessing, identifying, and implementing approaches, and evaluating results in relation to care of the ill or potentially ill person. (Jones 1977)†

This may sound long-winded, but it is very concise when compared with the job definition of the general practitioner (see p. 98).

The nursing process has four stages:

(1) assessment, problem identification and, in conjunction with patient, determination of goals;
(2) planning to achieve the agreed goals;
(3) implementation of measures decided upon;
(4) evaluation, and determination whether goals have been achieved.

It is a management process very similar to those described in this book, and having many points in common with the job definition of the general practitioner. This is as it should be; their goals in patient care should be the same. They share the same patient, and the same context. All that separates them is that they employ different, but complementary skills. Each interacts with the patient and with one another.

In the case quoted on p. 84, the doctor makes a provisional diagnosis and asks the district nurse to call – having given her some information. She makes an assessment based on information from several sources – doctor, relatives, health visitor, and her own observations. She identifies the nursing problem, sets her goals, and reports back to the general practitioner. Together with the patient and supporter they make a plan, and each plays his or her part in its implementation. Together, one hopes, they evaluate the success or otherwise of their efforts.

This is very different from the traditional approach, in which the doctor asks (or tells!) the nurse to do a bed bath or give an enema, treating the nurse as an inferior who takes orders, rather than a colleague and fellow-member of the team. A wider understanding of the nursing process by all practice staff will make co-operation easier, and co-ordinated care more effective.

†Jones, C. (1977). The nursing process – individualized care. *Nursing Mirror.* Oct. 13. pp. 13–14: quoted in *A new approach to district nursing* (1981). Ed. Monica Baly. Heinemann Medical Books.

6 Patients

Whether you look at general practice as a business, a caring profession, or an 'open system' †, patients are the prime concern – as customers, as people being cared for, or as 'input'. The practice manager does not need reminding of this everyday fact of life. Perhaps this should have been the first chapter in the book – it is certainly one of the most important from the viewpoint of management.

WHAT IS A PATIENT?

First, are we clear what is meant by the term 'patient'? Does it mean someone who is ill or disabled? Many are caring for themselves, and do not see themselves as patients. Does it mean someone getting professional care from medical, paramedical, or fringe practitioners? This is the more common meaning – someone who is suffering, not only the illness, but from the conditions which society imposes in order to 'legitimize' an illness, to make it fit in with the rules. Doctors are trained (in hospital) to expect patients to be compliant – giving up a large slice of their autonomy in return for receiving medical and paramedical treatment. This means the doctor taking decisions with which the patient is expected to comply, or be labelled a 'bad patient'. Many people are reluctant to accept a 'sick role', with its implied dependency and loss of autonomy. They prefer to take some responsibility for their own health, and be involved in the decisions about it. If presented with a 'take it or leave it' attitude, many leave it. They default from treatment, or treat themselves. Sometimes the sick-role is forced upon them, when they are very ill, worried, or need a certificate. They may still resent the loss of independence and self-esteem which goes with keeping oneself healthy.

To what extent to doctors and nurses encourage dependency, and compliance, or encourage medical help when self-help would do as well or better? Is this not a part of the present scene of mounting workload and over-prescribing? Are we not all responsible for some of it? Workload, prescribing, and self-help are discussed further in Chapter 10.

The question we must all answer is: 'Do we see the patient as someone who comes cap-in-hand for a free and skilled service; or as someone who comes as an equal to discuss his problem with a professional, and to be advised rather

† See p. 226 (Chapter 16) for a definition and further discussion.

than told?'. There is much in common with the leadership styles described in Chapter 7.

Psychologists would see the first as a 'parent–child' relationship, and the second as an 'adult–adult' relationship (Harris 1973). Doctors who try to adopt the latter style come nearer to what is known as 'counselling'. This means listening, helping the other person to define their problem, to think up solutions, and to choose between them. This is the reverse of the authoritarian style of the doctor who says 'take this – it will make you better'.

Another meaning of the word 'patient' is commonly used in general practice, but less in the world outside – namely people on the NHS list of a general practitioner, that is, potential patients. So the term 'patient' can refer to almost all the population†, whether ill or not and whether seeing a doctor or not. Doctors think of patients as the people at risk of becoming ill whom they are under contract to see on request. But does the general practitioner feel responsible for them when they make no demands upon his time? This is an area of change and controversy. Some doctors feel a sense of caring for the whole of their flock, including those who do not attend. Such doctors are likely to be keen on prevention, or screening – on using their knowledge to look ahead in their patients' interest, now called 'anticipatory care'. The doctor may know about the importance of immunization, cervical screening, checking blood pressure, and so on, but does he ensure that all of his patients benefit from this knowledge? This topic is dealt with in Chapter 11.

DOCTORS' ATTITUDES TO PATIENTS

We have so far considered four ways of looking at 'the patient', which can be arranged in a spectrum according to the attitudes of doctors and staff, and to some extent of the patients themselves. But are not the moulds in which we try to cast patients set by the behaviour of the doctors, and the way they see their patients and their work – in truth their whole philosophy? A table of these practice philosophies and behaviours in relation to patients is given (Table 6.1), and the management implications are considered.

Type I suits the old-fashioned authoritarian doctor, who knows best but explains little. In exchange for what may be excellent technical care, he expects total obedience from the patient, who must do things his way. Many people are likely to opt out, and take themselves or be referred elsewhere.

Type II represents a more modern viewpoint where the doctor tries to practice 'whole-person medicine', even if the strain on his time and energy is severe. Doctors who practice a wider range of social and psychological problems themselves, rather than refer them to other agencies. They usually expect the manager to cope, and are perhaps less sensitive to the needs of the organization.

† Ninety-eight per cent of the population (Cartwright and Anderson 1981) but only 75 per cent in some inner cities.

Table 6.1. *Views about patients*

I	Ill people who accept doctor's advice and comply with treatment *Patient as pawn*	'Tells', 'authoritarian'
II	Ill people who attend and are free to negotiate about intervention by doctor *Patient as friend or equal*	'Counselling', 'consulting'
III	Whole practice population considered in terms of keeping well and preventing illness, by anticipatory care *Patient seen as ally in search of health*	'Goal-seeking', 'consulting'
IV	Whole practice population considered to be at risk, but only seen on request. Preventive action on request only *Patient may be seen as a nuisance or even an enemy*	'Laissez-faire'

Type III combines the doctor who deals with demand as it arises – perhaps more selectively and critically than the others – and who places more emphasis on improving his patients' health, even if they are not so keen. He will be an enthusiast for health education, but can only get away with it if he has earned his patients' respect by his caring and curing. He will put greater demands on management for developing systems and self-help groups (Chapter 10), age–sex registers and disease indexes (Chapter 11), and computers (Chapter 12).

Type IV is a more traditional viewpoint. The doctor takes what comes his way, and may be overwhelmed by workload. He makes no attempt to look ahead or manage. The practice manager may have a problem in trying to get a quart (of patients) into a pint pot (of appointments). She may try to protect him from overwork, so that patients become a nuisance and overdemanding, with 'trivial illnesses'. A practice which resists change can be very dispiriting, but the challenge to overcome the difficulties is all the greater.

Four kinds of doctor's behaviour and attitudes to patients

From the starting point of how patients are viewed, we end up with four kinds of behaviour. The picture is exaggerated and all varieties and mixtures are possible in a practice, even in a single doctor. But the message is clear – patients, policies, people, and management are all inextricably linked, and the spectrum of doctors' and patients' behaviour is very wide. To try to match the doctor's behaviour and attitudes to the patient's expectations and vice versa is a formidable task. The practice manager needs to understand the complexity of the process and the subtle influences at work, so that she can remove some of the barriers to communication, and set the scene for better doctor–patient rapport.

Figure 6.1 tries to clarify the types of attitude and behaviour seen in different doctors. Two of the stereotypes can be seen as being at opposite ends of a spectrum, with all gradations possible between the extremes. At right angles are the other two. On the right is Type I – the 'doctor-centred' and rather technical

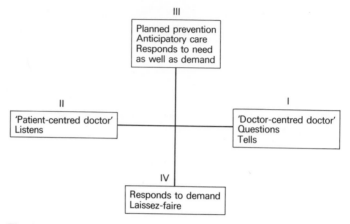

Fig. 6.1. Four kinds of attitude to patients and behaviour by doctors.

doctor, who asks questions and tells the patient how to get well. On the left is Type II – the 'patient-centred' doctor who listens and helps the patient to get himself well. These variations of behaviour have been described and studied by Byrne and Long (1976) in their classical work *Doctors talking to patients*, to whom the reader is referred for details.

At the top of the figure is the Type III doctor – interested in promoting health and preventing illness, rather than waiting for it to happen. This has been well described by Dr. Julian Tudor Hart (1981) as 'A new kind of doctor'. At the bottom of the figure (in more senses than one) is the doctor who responds only to demand and who may sink into apathy when the going is tough.

It is artificial to put people into definite categories, when one considers the wide range of behaviour, even in one individual. People change their behaviour to suit different circumstances, and have we not stressed before that learning is all about behavioural change?

An activity which should enliven a dull practice meeting would be to ask doctors to plot on Fig. 6.1 where they think they stand, and where they think their partners stand. If they felt really courageous they could ask the staff and patients where they would stick the flag!

LISTENING TO PATIENTS

Anyone who has observed what goes on at the reception hatch is impressed with the quantity of information which has to pass in both directions, and the number of decisions which have to be taken. Let us first consider the information from the patient.

From the moment the patient decides to seek help until he or she meets the doctor, the lines of communication will be under the practice manager's control. Are they adequate? Can patients speak freely at the hatch? Are receptionists trained to listen? What about people with different social or cultural backgrounds, different health beliefs, or language problems? (see Fuller and Toon 1988). Can they be given the opportunity to get their message across in privacy? Is an interview room needed for the receptionist? What about people who have hearing loss, or are not familiar with the telephone? Can the manager train and supervise staff so that they can cope? Does she undertake a counselling role with staff and patients when things go wrong? Some of these questions are considered in other chapters, but the practice manager may have to find the answers to all the questions, as best she can.

A particular problem is the difficult or aggressive patient. Often they have screwed up their courage to come to the surgery, and are expecting a particular outcome – such as seeing the doctor straight away. If their expectations are not met they may explode. Then, if the doctor appears, their manner changes to sweet reasonableness – a double blow for the receptionist or practice manager!

It may be helpful for the receptionists to note the names of patients whom they find difficult, for discussion at a meeting with the doctors. Often they are mentally ill or handicapped, or have severe social problems or difficulty in communicating. When the reason is made clear and discussed, the problem may disappear.

Patients' views and rights

The consumer movement is here to stay, and there is no reason why general practice should escape its attention. When patients speak about general practice it is against a background of approval for NHS care. Cartwright and Anderson (1981), in a detailed study of patients' attitudes, found that patients did not complain easily, and showed an 'uncritical acceptance and lack of discrimination which is conducive to stagnation and apathy'. In the 13 years between Cartwright's two studies, the criticism of 'failure to visit when asked' had increased fourfold, and that of 'failure to examine' twofold. Patients were critical of doctors' failure to listen and to explain things fully. They also criticized doctors who were relatively inaccessible.

Patients praised the doctor when he was good at discovering the patients' real concerns and expectations, and meeting them; when the doctor's manner communicated warmth, and interest in the patient; and when the doctor volunteered information which was explained in terms the patient could understand.

Pendleton's (1981) research has shown that patients are keen to be involved in making decisions about their health *with* the doctor. Only a few wanted an authoritarian doctor who told them what to do.

There is some evidence that patients now are better informed about health, and want to be treated in a more adult manner. Patients' expectations about treatment have risen, and they are more prepared to criticize.

The National Consumer Council has made a thorough study of patients' and doctors' rights and responsibilities in the NHS, and has published a small booklet (NCC 1982) which puts the case as fairly as possible. Every practice manager would be wise to have a copy, and make sure that receptionists are aware of the relevant sections. It can be obtained from local Community Health Council offices. The NCC also has summary leaflets which can be issued free to patients.

INFORMING PATIENTS

Patients absorb information about a surgery the minute they walk in. Is the atmosphere friendly? Do people smile at you? Are direction signs clear and notices helpful? Or is the place unwelcoming, and full of notices like 'don't bother the doctor, he's busy', so that patients feel unwanted and guilty about being ill?

Written information can be in the form of handouts about services available, with the names of doctors and staff, telephone numbers, and so on. This type of handout is considered in Chapter 8. Handouts about health education are considered in Chapter 12. But there is an intermediate area in which doctors and staff can state their aims and philosophy – that they believe in people keeping well, in looking after themselves if they can, but any help being easily available if they cannot; in preventing unnecessary illness by immunization, not smoking, etc. They can state that they do not believe in too much prescribing if it can be avoided (e.g. slimming pills, sleeping pills, cough mixtures). They can say that they like to work together as a team and that patients have access to all of them. Policy about personal doctoring and change of doctor can be set out. This sort of handout sets the scene for patients, and perhaps enables them to reveal their own expectations more clearly. As a result the relationship may be more open and more freely negotiated. Informing patients is part of the health education process, considered in Chapter 10. So far we have mostly considered the individual patient and his or her needs. What about the patients as a group and their collective needs and expectations?

THE PATIENT PARTICIPATION GROUP

Practices have been showing an increasing interest in this development since 1972. In 1981 the numbers of groups almost doubled, and growth is still rapid. There are many things patients will not say to the doctor in the consultation. They are anxious, do not want to upset the doctor, and time is short. But a representative group of users of the surgery or health centre, will – if given the chance – make constructive suggestions about improving the service, and will implement changes themselves. Examples of this have been the running of surgery car services, good neighbour groups, postnatal support groups, luncheon clubs for the elderly, prescription-collection services, practice newsletters, and so on. The achievements of these groups have been remarkable.

Though the doctors need to be sympathetic and show some enthusiasm to get things started, most of the energy comes from the patient group.

The types of activity come under eight main headings:

1, A dialogue between user and provider, so that some balance can be achieved between any conflicting aims and expectations.

2. Providing feedback for planning new services and evaluating existing ones.

3. Calling attention to gaps in services, and helping to fill the gaps if possible.

4. Co-ordinating existing community networks to improve health care.

5. Providing a forum for grumbles, complaints, and praise for both users and providers.

6. Encouraging and organizing health promotion, and educational activities appropriate to people's health beleifs and levels of understanding.

7. Providing resources of knowledge, skill, and energy to improve health through primary health care.

8. Being prepared to lobby outside bodies to improve the level or co-ordination of health care.

Accountability of general practitioners is largely missing in the NHS as organized at present, and there are strong moves to increase it through ombudsmen, complaints procedures, and charters of patients' rights. These all have a place in the system, but a meeting of doctors with a group of their patients in an atmosphere of mutual trust could well increase accountability as a trade-off for the very real help which a patient group gives to a practice. It provides the practice with a listening post in the community whose value cannot be exaggeraged.

Several practice managers have set up patient groups which have been successful. A practical guide has been published on how to set up a group (Pritchard 1983), to which reference can be made. A varied collection of essays has been published by the RCGP (1981a), and further information is available in Pritchard (1981; pp. 114–124). Patients are mentioned in every chapter of this book, but we now turn to the general practitioner's role in management.

Further reading

Information for patients.

Clayton, S. (1988). Information for patients. In: *Information handling in general practice* (eds. R. Jones and R. Westcott). Chapman and Hall, London.

Accountability

Pritchard, P. (1986). Professional accountability in general practice. In: *Medical Annual 1986*, (eds D. and J. Gray). Wright, Bristol.

Patient participation

Paine, T. (1987). How to do it — set up a patient participation group. *Br. Med. Jnl.* **295** 828–9.

7 The general practitioner's role in management

WHAT IS GENERAL PRACTICE?

The general practitioner's main job is diagnosis and treatment of his patients' illnesses. Management's major function is to support him in fulfilling his role. There is more to general practice than this simple statement, so it might be helpful to quote the definition of a general practitioner published by the Royal College of General Practitioners (RCGP 1972). This definition has since been modified by a European working party, but the original definition is preferred.

The doctor who provides personal, primary and continuing medical care to individuals and families. He may attend his patients in their homes, in his consulting-room or sometimes in hospital. He accepts the responsibility for making an initial decision on every problem his patient may present to him, consulting with specialists when he thinks it appropriate to do so. He will usually work in a group with other general practitioners, from premises that are built or modified for the purpose, with the help of paramedical colleagues, adequate secretarial staff and all the equipment which is necessary. Even if he is in single-handed practice he will work in a team and delegate when necessary. His diagnoses will be composed in physical, psychological and social terms. He will intervene educationally, preventively and therapeutically to promote his patient's health.

This definition of the doctor's role goes far beyond diagnosis and treatment. It includes:

referral to specialists;
working with other doctors;
purpose-built (or modified) premises;
secretarial staff;
all necessary equipment;
team working with nurses and others;
diagnosing in physical, psychological, and social terms;
education and prevention as well as treatment.

This list makes it clear that the general practitioner no longer works alone, as in the past. He has to be in charge of administrative staff and premises in support of his main role. He has to work with professional staff who have different training and aims, and who (like him) enjoy a high degree of autonomy – that is to say they make their own decisions; they do not take orders from doctors.

By extending the role to include psychological and social diagnoses he has to have a much wider information base than previously, as well as having to use his time more carefully. By including prevention and education, he extends his interest to people who do not call on his services spontaneously, and who are not necessarily ill at all.

WHAT IS PRIMARY HEALTH CARE?

The wider role of the general practitioner described here, places him firmly in the context of *primary health care*, which is the more appropriate term to cover the work of the whole team.

So what is primary health care, and how does it differ from general practice as described above? Whereas general practice, by tradition, is mainly concerned with treatment of disease presented by 'patients', the emphasis in primary health care is on *health* and its promotion by a healthy life style, by prevention of ill health if possible, and by the provision of acceptable first-line health care to which all people have access, and which they can afford.

This alteration in emphasis is strongly supported by the World Health Organization† (WHO), which has found by experience that this is a better way of improving people's health, than the old style emphasis on treating illness – important as it is.

The WHO has also concluded that for primary health care to flourish and improve people's health, certain requirements must be met:

1. Health care must be related to people's needs.

2. Consumers should participate individually and collectively in the planning and implementation of health care.

3. Fullest use must be made of existing resources, which implies good co-operation between health and other sectors such as employment, social services, and housing.

4. Primary health care must be integrated with secondary and tertiary care (i.e. hospitals and super-specialties).

5. There must be proper support for management, for education, and for research based on primary health care.

6. The overriding requirement is for adequate financial support of primary health care, which will not happen without a firm political will that it should succeed.

These topics are discussed further in Chapter 18.

---

† The World Health Assembly has ratified the aim of achieving optimum health for all by the year 2000, through the development of primary health care, both in developing and in industrialized countries (WHO/UNICEF 1978; Kaprio, 1979).

HOW HEALTHY IS THE NATIONAL HEALTH SERVICE?

What has all this got to do with managing general practice? It sets the scene, so that we can assess the national policies and strategies within which we have to work, and how priorities are assessed and selected. Governments and administrations have to manage effectively and efficiently or the 'first-line' caring role is made much more difficult. So first let us ask ourselves how the National Health Service (NHS) in the United Kingdom measures up to the WHO yardsticks.

Relating health care to need

The NHS is very 'demand-orientated', and this is fine, provided that substantial groups are not being left out and that money is not being wasted. Alas, there are many underserved groups such as the elderly, the mentally handicapped, people who do not register with a doctor, or those who fail to attend when ill (see Hannay 1979). Money is invested in high-technology hospital care, leaving less for primary health care.

Consumer involvement in planning and implementation

The NHS record is good, with a Community Health Council for every district (a unique achievement which other countries applaud) and increasing emphasis on patient participation at individual and practice level. But planning is still largely dominated by professional aims without due regard for the aims and aspirations of the consumers, as reports of Community Health Councils will confirm.

Co-operation between health and other sectors

We have not yet achieved the co-ordinated provision of care between, for example, health and social services. Each pursues its own aims and philosophies with little thought for the other. Sometimes good local co-operation can be worked out, but lack of national policy and a common administrative framework make for muddle rather than efficiency.

Integration of primary health care with hospital care

For historical reasons, medicine has been dominated by the teaching hospitals, and GPs are still the by-product rather than the end-product of medical education. The teaching of medicine is largely based on the very small proportion of patients admitted to teaching hospitals, by referral paths which are not properly understood.

Support for management education and research based on primary health care

The picture is changing, with mandatory vocational training for general practitioners, health visitors, and district nurses, but practice manager training is only just gaining momentum. Management support for primary health care lags far behind that provided for hospitals.

Financial support for primary health care

In spite of Government policy statements about supporting primary health care, it has been receiving a relatively smaller share of the NHS funds in recent years. Only a strong political commitment to the development of primary health care will ensure that policies become realities.

Though the NHS can claim a better record than most other industrialized countries, we cannot be very satisfied about the way it measures up to the yardstick described above. One difficulty is that the performance of primary health care, or of general practice, cannot be clearly measured, so we do not really know how well or badly we are doing. Without clear policies and aims for general practice, and measures of success, we have difficulty in competing for funds.

As a first stage, we must accept that we live in an imperfect world, and must make our plans accordingly. But making the best use of present constraints may help to improve the system locally. If enough people act in the same way, the pressure for change will build up. The NHS has improved in a number of ways since 1948, and much of this has been due to pressure from below. Though it is a 'top-down' system of planning and control, there are elements of 'bottom-up' planning – where ideas generated locally are accepted centrally. The ideal solution is integrated planning at all levels and it is hoped that the new (April 1982) District Health Authorities will be a move in this direction. Plans will work only if general practitioners try to work together to achieve agreed aims, and provide an input into planning through membership of authorities, planning teams, advisory committees, etc. The general practitioners' independent contractor status has helped him to retain his professional autonomy in the face of an expanding bureaucracy, but too much autonomy can lead to an uneven service to patients. There has been evidence of this in inner cities, and public disquiet about the quality of general practice is increasing. More detailed consideration of planning can be found in Chapter 17.

COPING WITH CHANGE

So far we have considered the broader picture of the NHS, and the implications for primary health care. It is not a static picture, but is changing all the time. Many changes are occurring within general practice, but most changes that affect us come from outside the practice. We can have more control of internal changes, but must adapt to external changes if we are to survive. Any linking mechanisms which may help the process of adaptation are important, and are listed separately.

Each practice and each community is unique in the range of changes affecting it, though some broad generalizations can be made. A list of changes now affecting most practices is given below, but it is better for each practice to construct its own list.

Factors for change within general practice

Spread of vocational training;
increasing interest in performance review (audit);
increasing interest in prevention of ill-health;
increasing interest in computers;
increasing interest in team working;
more management education for GPs and staff;
more practice managers in post;
more practice nurses in post;
more attached nursing staff;
social-skills training in consultation;
spread of patient participation groups;
more female general practitioners;
development of community hospital concept;
workload changing, (?) increasing;
more effective treatments available in general practice.

Factors for change from outside general practice

Medical

Financial cuts in NHS—cash limits;
fewer hospital beds;
shorter hospital stay;
emphasis on community care;
longer waiting time in certain areas;
super-specialization, and high-technology.

Social

Population changes † – numbers, age structure, family size, and ethnic mix;
decreased spending by local authorities on social services;
changing expectations of health and social care;
increasing unemployment;
technical advances in coping with disability.

Mechanisms linking the practice and the outside world

Clinical assistantships in hospital;
special clinics in general practice (e.g. diabetic);
extended team work;
self-help groups;
health education;
patient participation group;
membership of management team, etc.

† In the past 20 years, the numbers of people over 65 have risen by one-third. They now constitute 15 per cent of the population. By the end of the century the number aged 75 and over will have increased by one-third, and the number aged 85 and over by one-half.

Table 7.1. Predicting change and planning ahead

Factors for change	1974	1980	1981	1982	1983	1984	1985	1986	2000	Comments
List population	8500	9000	9500	10000	10400	10800	11200	11500	12000	
List 65–74		800		900				1000	1100	
75 and over		550		600				760	920	
85 and over				220					330	
Partners	3	3	4	4	4	5	5	5½	6	
Trainee	–	–	1	1	1	1	1	2	2	
Staff employed WTE	4½	4½	6*	6	6½	7½	7½	8	9	*Practice manager started in 1981
Staff attached WTE	2½	3	3	3	3½	3½	4	5 + 1†	6 + 1	†Application for FT attached social worker in 1986
Clinical work, etc.			Diabetic clinic		Counsellor	Prevention programme	Geriatric survey			
Systems and equipment			Age–sex register	Disease index	A4 notes	Computer	New†† ECG		Extend computer	††Original ECG bought 1975
Outside appointments	2	2	3	3	3	4	5	5	6	
Education and training			1st GP trainee	Receptionist training	In-house staff training	Practice nurse training	Partners sabbatical leave	2nd GP trainee		
Premises			Added on two consulting suites	New estate completed		Portakabin in car park		Move to new centre		
Community		Self help groups			Start patient group	Surgery car service				

WTE = whole-time equivalent staff; FT = full-time; ECG = electrocardiograph machine.

Looking to the future

Listing changes gives a 'snapshot' of a given time, but does not indicate the rate of change. This can be achieved by making a table of past changes and trying to anticipate the future. Just as each practice must make its own list of factors for change, so must the table be constructed by each practice. An example is given in Table 7.1, which follows an idea presented by Dr. Peter Havelock.

Devising such a table is a useful and entertaining exercise. The figures for past list sizes can be obtained from the quarterly statement of fees and allowances sent by the Family Practitioner Committee. Once the age-sex register is completed, a figure could be obtained for patients aged 85 and over, which would show an even more dramatic increase by the year 2000. Help with population projections could be obtained from the Planning Officer of the District Health Authority or the Community Physician. The practice shown has a future growth rate of 2.5 per cent per annum, but there is no measure of population turnover (which generates much extra work). This figure can be obtained from the FP 22A forms listing weekly removals.

Decisions about taking on a new partner or a trainee, or changes to premises need to be planned well ahead. Similarly the purchase of the computer needs to be tied in with the prevention programme and engaging extra staff (see Chapter 12).

If all the staff concerned can be involved in making the table, they will be encouraged to think to the future, and to plan it together. It can provide a powerful stimulus to nursing management to budget for an adequate establishment of attached district nurses and health visitors. A table such as this provides a series of targets, and progress towards them can be monitored and the targets revised if necessary.

We have been considering one way of responding to change. There are others:

Responses to change

1. Ignore it – it can't happen here!
2. Respond passively when forced to.
3. Predict likely changes and plan ahead (as in Table 7.1).
4. Actively pursue and bring about favourable changes – 'inventing the future'.

The last two methods require enthusiasm, energy, and foresight; and the determination to overcome apathy (or even downright hostility). Fortunately these are qualities with which GPs and practice managers are well endowed. People do not like change, unless they are involved in its planning, and can see some advantage for themselves. A summary of suggestions for implementing change is given below.

Guidelines for implementing change

1. Discuss the need for change.
2. Make a thorough diagnosis before deciding on treatment.

3. Make clear plans.
4. Discuss plans with all the people involved, and amend if necessary.
5. Make a timetable – be flexible.
6. Monitor progress – watch out for backlash.
7. People may resist change because:
    (a) they are anxious or threatened – discuss and reassure (facts help);
    (b) they are apathetic – may need a prod;
    (c) they are confused – discuss and clarify;
    (d) there is nothing in it for them – re-plan so that there is.

8. Remember that change should not be just an exercise of power; nor is it a rational process – it involves people and feelings.

9. Change is a process of mutual learning and problem-solving, which may not necessarily end you up where you planned to go initially!

The last guideline reminds us to ask ourselves an important question.

WHERE ARE WE HEADING?

How often do we ask ourselves what we are trying to achieve? What are our objectives? In broad terms they can be stated as:

1. Providing first-line health care which is *accessible* to the whole population.
2. Providing an *acceptable* level and quality of service.
3. Identifying those health needs of the population which can be prevented, modified, or treated.
4. Making optimum use of manpower and resources to meet the health needs of the population – including promotion of a healthy lifestyle, preventive, and curative services.

(modified from Marson *et al.* 1973)

These are broad aims. † To put them into action requires much more detail. When we start to make detailed objectives we meet several problems. Some objectives run counter to one another, for example, spending too much time on objectives 1 and 2 leaves no time for 3 and 4. So we have to make choices between desirable alternatives and this means drawing up priorities.

It is helpful to work out objectives, and try to write them down. Each one prompts four questions:

1. What are we trying to achieve? (e.g. a 100 per cent immunization rate).
2. How do we achieve it? (e.g. an efficient register and recall system).
3. How do we know if and when we have achieved it? (e.g. check the register at stated intervals).
4. Will this objective clash with others, and how will priorities be determined?

---

† Aims, goals, objectives. These words are often used interchangeably. They all mean 'a preferred outcome in a particular situation' (Beishon and Peters 1981). Objectives can be short-term to long-term; achievable to unachievable; measurable to unmeasurable. They can to some extent be put in an order (or hierarchy) from the very long-term (less achievable and less measurable) to the very short-term (more clearly achievable and checkable).

It is difficult for the general practitioner to work out a detailed 'hierarchy of objectives'. The practice manager can pave the way, but she needs the co-operation of the doctors and other staff to decide on priorities and criteria – particularly if they have to alter their behaviour (e.g. check a patient's blood pressure if there is a red 'flag' in the notes). A more detailed discussion of objectives appears in Pritchard (1981, pp. 12–22).

Whose objectives?

GPs, as independent contractors, 'own' the business side of their practice, which may include substantial capital assets. They are the board of directors, perhaps with the senior partner as chairman and managing director. It is natural for them to think that they 'own' the objectives too. This is a short-sighted view, as other people are usually involved in carrying out the objectives. The other people – lay staff, nurses, patients – may have other aims which are incompatible with those of the doctors. Unless there is some awareness of these other aims, and some measure of consultation and compromise, failure is certain. So doctors must ask themselves more questions in addition to the first one – 'what are the doctors' aims?':

Are the doctors' aims shared by other staff – professional and lay?
What are the staff's aims?
What aims and aspirations do patients have in relation to general practice?
Can all these aims be reconciled?
How?

THE GENERAL PRACTITIONER AS MANAGER

Several areas of practice management have been described in which the general practitioner has a unique part to play. These include:

defining his role;
coping with change;
planning the future;
helping to formulate objectives;
deciding on priorities.

Does he accept these as part of his function? Assuming the answer is 'yes', the next questions are:

How does he manage – what is his style?
How does he lead?
How are decisions made?
Once made, are decisions implemented?

Styles of management

Different people manage in different ways according to their personality, age and experience. Likert (1967) has described four: Exploitive – authoritative;

benevolent – authoritative; consultative; and participative – group. To which of these stereotypes do doctors liken themselves – or their colleagues? Would they have the courage to ask their staff which picture fits them? By involving other people, the last two styles are more likely to be successful, but there are moments of crisis when authority has to be exercised.

The general practitioner as leader

Some doctors may be reluctant to manage, or there may be agreement that one doctor is managing director. Alternatively, different parts of the practice may be managed by different partners, e.g. staff, team, buildings, education, communication, prevention, computerization. Whether or not they manage, all doctors have to be leaders, as do practice managers and health visitors, in their own field. It is expected that they should take a lead, though that does not mean that they have to be bossy all the time!

Leadership style is a continuum between extreme authoritarianism at one end and freedom for subordinates at the other end; this range of possible behaviour is shown in Fig. 7.1. This is not a scale from leadership to non-leadership but a gradation in ways of leading. Where does the reader see himself on this scale, and where do his colleagues or subordinates see him?

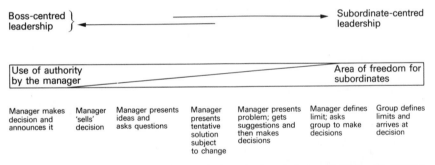

Fig. 7.1. Continuum of leadership behaviour. (From Tannenbaum and Schmidt (1958).) Note: The seven categories of behaviour shown above are almost identical with the categories used by Byrne and Long (1976) in describing general practitioners' behaviour in the consultation. The main differences are that the order has been reversed, with the more authoritarian behaviour on the right, and there is a whole extra category of authoritarian behaviour beyond the one shown here!

For those who are not at home with 'power-shift diagrams' it may be preferable to describe three styles of leadership. The 'Tells' style represents the extreme left of the continuum, the 'Consulting' style the extreme right, and the 'Laissez-faire' style somewhere off the page (see Table 7.2).

Ways of looking at leadership, and of assessing its quality are considered further in Chapter 18.

Table 7.2. *Three styles of leadership*

'Tells' style of leadership
   Only one brain
   Task oriented
   Lack of creative thinking
   People treated as robots
   Constant supervision
   No joint discussion/decision making
   Work allocated by boss
   Job satisfaction tends to be low

'Consulting' style of leadership
   Discusses problems/involves the group
   Joint decision making
   Work allocation left more to the members themselves
   All brains are used
   Creative thinking encouraged
   People feel as if they are wanted
   Job satisfaction tends to be high
   High morale
   Boss approachable
   Work gets done well and effectively

'Laissez-faire' style of leadership
   Inconsistent leadership
   Boss difficult to pin down
   Work group have to fend for themselves
   Work group tend to elect their own leader
   (But he has no authority outside the group)
   Boss not trusted by the group
   Tendency towards low morale
   Tends not to be task-oriented
   Work not co-ordinated
   Work not completed
   Leader seen as being irresponsible

DECISION-MAKING

General practitioners and staff work in an area of great uncertainty. Information may be scanty, communication may be faulty, and time may be short. But 'he has to make an initial decision on every problem his patient may present to him'. By and large doctors are quite good at solving problems and making decisions about patients. Observation shows that they are less good at making decisions about the practice. Some doctors avoid decisions at all cost, lest conflict should ensue; others fail to apply the 'diagnosis before treatment' model which works well with patients. Can we provide some guidelines which will help decision-making in the practice?

It would be nice to think that decision-making could be described as a clear, logical process without any uncertainty. This is rarely so, but can happen in circumstances where an algorithm or decision treee is applicable. An example is shown on p. 122. To follow it, questions have to be asked in the right order, and the answer comes out at the end. All the alternatives have to be considered, and decisions taken in constructing the algorithm, so the person following it hardly has to decide anything. Computers can be programmed to interact in a similar way.

Decisions are affected by emotions and beliefs, as well as by information and logic. How can we take them all into account? The following check list is taken from Drucker (1974):

1. What is the decision about?
2. Is there need for a decision?
3. Can we all agree on that, rather than jump to solutions on which we disagree?
4. What information do we have, and is it fact or opinion?
5. What alternatives are available?
6. What limiting factors are there?
7. What compromises are available?
8. Can we obtain feedback on the successes or otherwise of the decision?

Having considered the problem and ways it might be solved, we can move to action which can be summarized:

consider (as above);
consult – information, ideas, opinion;
generate alternatives;
choose – i.e. decide what, who, how, when;
inform of decision;
check result against aims.

A more detailed check-list for decision-making can be obtained from the British Institute of Management, Parker Street, London WC2B 5PT (Management Check List No. 19).

Decisions should be recorded, both in the minutes of meetings (see Chapter 3) and also in a decision book. This makes it easier to check if action has been taken and what the result has been. Some decisions may cover future actions, and are codified as practice policies or rules.

POLICIES AND RULES

Whenever decisions have to be made between alternatives, the question must be asked 'is this an isolated occasion on which a specific decision is needed?' If not, then much time can be saved by having a *practice policy* covering each class of decision. In general, policies must be decided by the partners, after consulting the people concerned, but implementation of policies can be carried out at other levels, e.g. by the practice manager, or the receptionists. Then the partners need be bothered only if there is a decision to be made not covered by policy. If the new decision is likely to be a recurrent one, then it can be made a matter of policy. Policies are more essential in larger practices, but even in small practices staff change and misunderstandings occur, for which policies may be helpful. They must be recorded in the practice Decisions/Policy book, and kept up-to-date and reviewed as circumstances demand. This is a proper function of the practice manager. With this book to back her up, it is easier for her to carry out her mediating role, and to train new staff.

Written statements of policy help a practice to define its philosophy, from which strategies and plans can flow. If this philosophy is unclear, or different partners are working to different philosophies, then problems will arise. This is not to say that all partners must think alike; but they must know in which areas they agree, and in which they do not. Many partnerships are unhappy because individuals have diametrically opposing views – about patients' care, or about innovation, for example. It is possible that clear statements of policy could isolate the conflict to a smaller area, and not let it sour all the working relationships. Indeed, a new partner joining a practice would be greatly helped if he had the opportunity to see the practice policies, as he does the practice accounts.

In summary, practice policies help to:

(1) define practice philosophy and values;
(2) provide the basis for practice strategies and plans;
(3) maximize the areas of agreement;
(4) define 'forbidden territory';
(5) provide guidelines for delegated action;
(6) increase practice effectiveness.

All practices have policies, though mostly they are unrecorded, and often unspoken. To be fully effective they must be written down. The policies are unique to each practice, so no model policy document is possible but some guidance might be helpful in this formidable task. The process of formalizing policies is a valuable learning experience for the practice. A check-list of areas in which policies might be needed is given in Table 7.3.

Table 7.3. *Practice policies: A check-list of possible areas*

Acceptance of patients
  Geographical area of practice
  Accepting patients outside area
  Any selective acceptance of patients approved?
  List of numbers and closure of certain partner's lists
  Accepting patients from other practices
Patient procedures
  Personal lists
  Changing doctors within practice
  Procedures for new patients (e.g. information, interview, screening)
  Certification
Accessibility
  Flexibility of session to meet demand
  Appointment procedures
  Urgent appointments
  Home visit requests
  Access by telephone to doctor

Prevention and health promotion
    At-risk groups screened
    Health education for individuals and groups
    Self-help groups

Prescribing
    Repeat prescription procedures (prescribing policies would be listed under Clinical policies)

Communication
    With: staff;
            attached staff (team working);
            hospitals and other outside organizations;
            patients;
            organizations in the community
    Confidentiality

Staff
    Numbers of staff
    Job specifications
    Selection
    Training
    Delegation procedures
    Holidays and sick leave
    Discipline
    Amenities

Premises and equipment
    Maintenance and decoration

Partners
    Future size of practice
    Number of outside sessions
    Equalizing workload/case load
    Night and weekend rotas
    Manning the telephone
    Use of deputizing service or locums
    Holidays. Study leave
    Covering for trainee
    Retirement age

Finance
    Balance between income and practice expenses
    Partners' shares and drawings
    Private fees and outside sessions
    Seniority and other allowances
    Charges to patients
    Financial control and budget delegation

The distinction has been made already between practice management and the management of patients with diseases. Similarly, there are practice policies covering the running of the practice, including services for patients; and there are purely clinical policies – say for the care of diabetic patients. Both are essential, and interdependent, but the emphasis here is on the practice policies. For a very clear exposition of these topics see Buckley, E. G. (1982). Practice policy. *British Medical Journal* **285**, 177–9, and Clinical policies, *British Medical Journal* **285**, 351–2.

Rules

Rules are less important, and are usually internal administrative matters. They still need to be decided upon after consultation and reviewed, or they will not be kept. They come in three varieties:

(1) formal;
(2) informal;
(3) personal.

Formal rules are agreed and written, and overlap with policies. They might cover such things as routine reception tasks and communication of messages.

Informal rules are unwritten, and arise as 'this is the way we do things here'. They can vary from the highest code of ethical behaviour to 'how we refuse requests for visits' – which may be against practice policies. In a small closely-knit and highly-motivated practice, informal rules may be enough. However, they make life difficult for a new member of staff, and result in lax supervision and control of delegation.

There is an even more cryptic category – personal rules. Each doctor may have his own rules which he tells the receptionist but no one else. Or she may learn of them the hard way by his behaviour if she tries to fit in another patient, or put through a phone call. The fewer personal rules the better. Firmness and tact from the practice manager may bring them out into the light of day, and turn them into more flexible, but formal rules.

We have seen that coping with change and decision-making are both a process of learning and compromise, involving a variety of different people and attitudes. More attention will be given to planning and problem-solving in Chapters 16 and 17, but let us now look briefly at legal constraints, and the important topic of management of time.

THE GENERAL PRACTITIONER AND THE LAW

Mention has been made of statutes covering employment and equal opportunity. Partnership agreements are essential legal documents which codify certain practice policies (e.g. about partnership shares). It is more important that the partnership agreement does accurately reflect the partners' policies, and is not a relic of a bygone age when the main aim of the agreement was to preserve the goodwill of the practice which had a cash value.

The practice manager may need to be familiar with legal issues facing general practice. They are usually well covered in publications like *Medeconomics* and *Pulse*. However, a legal textbook in the library is essential. The following are recommended:

Leahy Taylor, J. (1982). *Medical malpractice*, 2nd edn. Pitman, London.
Knight, B. (1987). *Legal aspects of medical practice*, 4th edn, Churchill Livingstone, Edinburgh.

MANAGEMENT OF TIME

Time is a precious commodity for the GP and practice staff. We all share the experience of being short of time to do all the things we would like to do. Is this a real shortage, and inevitable, or can good planning help us to make optimum use of the time available?

Different ways of viewing time

Time can be seen as a box of fixed dimensions, in which we try to cram our activities, as a commodity to be hoarded or spent like money, or as a measuring gauge which we cannot control. Alternatively, we can ignore the constraints of time and concentrate on achieving objectives in priority order, until time runs out.

Time as a box was neatly described by Professor C. Northcote Parkinson in his first 'law', that 'work expands to fill the time available for its completion'. In other words, we can always pad out the box so that it seems full, and then everyone is happy and feels useful. A corollary is the oft-quoted suggestion that if you want something done 'ask a busy man'. He knows how to pack the box more tightly.

Time as a commodity finds expression in phrases like 'spending time', 'saving time', or 'time budgeting'. But it is a less flexible commodity than money. Time cannot be put in the bank; it ticks away steadily, and is lost if not spent usefully. Time spent now may save time later, so the concept of 'investing' time in better organization and planning, and review is a valuable one which is referred to later.

But time shares with money the concept that what matters is not the rate of spending, or the total spent, but the value of the goods or services obtained with it. Value for money or cost-effectiveness is mirrored as 'time-effectiveness'. How effectively we do our work is a constant theme of this book, with time as the context.

The patient's view of time

Time is equally important for the patient, though the emphasis is often on the general practitioner being a busy person whose time is more precious. Patients like being seen as soon as possible, on their own assessment of urgency. They prefer not to be kept waiting when they come for an appointment, and they value greatly the doctor who seems to have plenty of time to listen, and deal with all their problems. They do not like the doctor who keeps looking at his watch, yet time is ticking away for the patient too.

It is remarkable that surveys have shown how many doctors manage to seem unhurried, when they are clearly 'working against the clock'. So time can seem a friend for the patient, but an enemy for the doctor. Patients are usually aware that the doctor is busy, and that they should not waste his time, so there is often a tacit agreement to end the consultation after the average 'six minutes for the patient'. This has become the norm in the NHS, whereas in North America it is common for the doctor to spend 20 or 30 minutes with each patient, and to be well rewarded financially for doing so. So let us consider how the doctor in the UK spends his time.

How do doctors spend their time?

Many surveys have been done about how GPs spend their time, † and a common factor is the wide variability. Some doctors have large lists, some have small; some doctors have high consultation rates, some do not; some doctors spend long hours in surgery or doing home visits, and some spend more time in ways other than seeing patients. It is very difficult to put a 'good' or 'bad' label on these activities. Doctors with large lists may be efficient, and have satisfied patients. High consultation rates may imply not a sensitivity to patient demand, but a failure of decision-making or planning of treatment. Time outside the consulting room may be used for planning, evaluation, team work, and prevention, and in many chapters of this book doctors and practice managers are urged to 'invest' time in these activities, with the implication that this will 'pay dividends' in more effective patient care and better health for all. The clear message is that the doctor who is a slave to demand will not be in a position to provide as effective a service, as the doctor who achieves a balance between meeting demand and planning ahead; between serving the patient directly or servicing the organization which serves the patient. To some extent this balance is affected by the philosophy of the doctor or the practice. To some extent it reflects the system of care and remuneration. It is no surprise that the North American family physician, who may spend eight hours or more daily in seeing patients in his office, is less concerned with prevention, care of the elderly or social aspects of health care. By contrast, the NHS general practitioner on average spends about half a day seeing patients, so has greater potential for other ways of providing primary health care. There are many different factors at work, so it is hard to compare like with like – however, such comparisons help us to broaden our horizons, and look afresh at the way we work.

The doctor who is not trapped in the treadmill of high demand is free to choose how to spend the remaining time. Will time be invested in efficient organization and control, in ways of forestalling demand by improving patients' health and helping them to use services more effectively, and in improving skills of doctors and staff?

Can we 'manage' time?

As mentioned above, it is how we spend our time that matters; we cannot control the passage of time. Efficient use of time means efficient management

---

† Hull, F. M. (1983). The GPs use of time: an international comparison. *Update* **26**, 1243–53. This excellent study shows that the average GP in the UK spends less than 13 per cent of his time in consultation (i.e. less than 25 hours per week). His Canadian counterpart nearly doubles that figure.

Table 7.4. *Check list of questions about management of time*†

1. Goals and policies
   Are the practice goals and policies clear?
   Is the practice, or are individual members trying to do too much?

2. Overload of time
   Are we working too many hours for optimum effectiveness?

3. Overload of tasks
   Are we doing too many jobs at once, or being interrupted too often?

4. Organization of work
   Do we plan ahead or wait for crises?
   Do we allot priorities, and try to do tasks in order of priority?
   Can the nature of the task be modified in order to save time? Does it have to be done at all?
   Is time wasted by bad co-ordination (e.g. late appointments or missing records)?
   Can the work be concentrated in a time of day at which the individual works best?
   Is effective use made of lists, diaries, planners etc?
   Is time allocated, where possible, or just left to chance?
   Is a margin of time and energy kept in reserve for contingencies?

5. Time off
   Are rest periods, days off, holidays and sabbaticals planned rationally?

6. Environment
   Is noise and distraction kept to a minimum?
   Can the telephone be made an ally, not a menace?

7. Attitude to work and to oneself
   Do we enjoy crises?
   Do we employ time-wasting practices?
   Are meetings used to waste time?
   Are we addicted to work for its own sake, or as a way of doing tasks?

†With acknowledgement to S. Otto.

of our work, so that we do not need to be too obsessed with time. If objectives are clearly formulated and understood, and priorities settled, time should – in a perfect world – look after itself. In reality what can we do to help? The first step is to discover how we spend our time. This means a study akin to a time and motion study in a factory. Help in mounting such a study can be sought from the Management Services Unit of the local health authority. Fatigue causes people to slow down by introducing time-wasting rituals, whereas a five minute break every hour to relax might forestall this. Time in meetings can be budgeted, by allowing time for each item in relation to its importance. Consulting times can be monitored unobtrusively, and doctors can study video tapes of their consultations to observe any time-wasting rituals. Alternatives to consultations can be explored – such as a telephone-time for follow-ups, or postal follow-up. A critical look can be taken of which activities need a doctor, and which can be delegated. Does the practice need a clinical psychologist, counsellor, a social worker, or a voluntary service organizer?

Delays in the system can be studied, e.g.

date and time appointment requested;
date and time of appointment;
time patient seen;
waiting time to see practice nurse;
delay time in arriving at a diagnosis;
waiting time for hospital investigations, appointments, etc.

The practice manager's role

The process of observing critically how time is spent is a form of 'action research' from which lessons are learned and corrective action taken. Such observation takes time, so an effort is needed to get the momentum going. The practice manager is in a key position to observe and study how time is spent, and she has a responsibility to hold the balance between the patients' and the organization's needs. If she is to 'manage' the doctors' time, she must ensure first that she manages her own time effectively.

A check-list on the management of time, applicable to all staff, is given in Table 7.4.

Further reading

Austin, B. (1979). *Time the essence. A manager's workbook for using time effectively.* British Institute of Management. Two small booklets which give a self-training programme for the keen manager.

British Institute of Management. Check list No. 1. *Effective use of executive time.* From British Institute of Management, Parker Street, London WC2B 5PT.

Bradley, N. C. A. (1983). Time and the general practice consultation. *The medical annual. Year book of general practice.* Wright PSG, Bristol. A good review with 37 references.

Reynolds, H. and Tramel, M. (1979). *Effective time management.* Gower Publishing. Aldershot. A well-written step-by-step approach.

Section B

Services and systems

8 Reception of patients

The reception service is the point of entry for people needing the care of the general practitioner and primary care team. It is also the way in to nearly all the other NHS services and many other agencies as well. The importance of a humane and efficient reception service cannot be stressed too much. Patients and staff are all dependent on its successful operation. Yet it is one area which is often criticized with terms such as the 'dragon at the gate', suggesting that there is a barrier to obtaining service, and that the dragon is there to defend the 'ogre in the castle'. Such terms live on, long after their justification has ended, but they are a warning to doctors and practice managers to check on their policies, procedures, and rules for this key area.

Reception of patients is not just a matter for receptionists; they can work only within the policies, framework, and resources laid down by the doctors and mediated by the practice manager. So the efficiency and effectiveness of the reception service reflects the philosophy and organization of the whole practice, as well as the selection and training of the individual receptionist, and the demands made by the population served. Practice policies, and selection and training have been discussed in previous chapters. How can all these elements be put together to ensure that the best possible service is provided?

OBJECTIVES

First we must be clear about the aims of a reception service. Is it to ensure a steady flow of patients to the doctor, one every six minutes, for the duration of the surgery session? Is it to meet all possible patient demand, however inconvenient for doctors and staff? As usual, it is a compromise between meeting all reasonable needs and expectations of patients, and the efficient use of the doctors' and nurses' time.

Accessibility

Accessibility is a major aim of primary health care, without which the service breaks down. Studies such as that made for the Royal Commission on the Health Service concluded that, on the whole, access is satisfactory.[†] Many factors govern access, some of which are outside the control of the practice, so

[†] HMSO (1979). *Access to primary care*. Research paper No. 6. Royal Commission on the Health Service, London.

allowance has to be made. Examples of factors affecting ease of access are listed below:

(1) possession of a telephone;
(2) availability of car transport, either patient's own car or a surgery car service;
(3) availability of public transport;
(4) mothers with small children – in particular single parents;
(5) distance between home and surgery or centre;
(6) patient's working hours, and ease of getting time off to see the doctor;
(7) unfamiliarity with the practice arrangements;
(8) cultural or language barriers;
(9) number of consulting hours per day in relation to list size;
(10) flexibility of consulting hours to meet peaks of demand;
(11) efficiency of monitoring of work load;
(12) procedures for dealing with urgent requests;
(13) practice policies about coping with work load, home visiting, accepting phone calls when consulting.

Some patients can cope with a barrier to access, while others, particularly those with less awareness that their problem might be urgent, may suffer. Patients who are ill or anxious may become aggressive, or give up the unequal struggle. All these factors reinforce the very difficult task which receptionists have to face, which they can only achieve satisfactorily when working to a well-designed system with the full support of doctors, other staff, and patients. Deciding what is a reasonable level of service or expectation can be helped by discussion with a group of patients.

The practice can exert little influence on many of the factors listed, but those subject to influence or control are considered further.

POLICIES

Practice policies about consulting hours, not refusing appointments, total numbers on list, locums to cover partners' absence, limiting practice area, and so on are of critical importance to accessibility. The whole practice philosophy – whether patients are regarded as a nuisance, or are treated with sympathy and kindness – will affect the way the reception service operates. Patients soon detect that a practice has a friendly welcoming atmosphere, and that they do not have to fight their way in.

STRUCTURE

The layout of the reception lobby and the design of the hatch are important. Patients and receptionists must have quiet and privacy. They must be able to make eye contact at about the same level, but not be so close to one another that they feel threatened. The appointment book must keep the names of attenders private. A separate interview room or area with greater privacy for patients who are distressed or deaf, or have confidential information, is an advantage. The telephone must be near to hand but not too intrusive, and it should not be possible for conversations to be overheard by third parties. Clear signposting, and the absence of distracting notices will help new patients.

PROCEDURES

It is helpful for receptionists to have procedures to cover all eventualities, so that they do not have to make decisions which may be upsetting or dangerous to the patient, or which depend on the exercise of medical knowledge. These can be written out at length (for an example see Pritchard (1981) *Manual of primary health care,* pp. 136–7). Such procedures should be reached by agreement, and regularly discussed and updated or they will be ignored. It may be useful for certain parts of the procedure to be in the form of an algorithm or decision-tree (see Fig. 8.1). Such a method is easy for beginners to refer to, and its construction helps to produce a logical sequence of behaviour, which saves effort.

Receptionists have to concentrate, and to 'give out' nearly all the time. This (as doctors and nurses find too) is exhausting. It has been shown that receptionists become less 'empathic', avoid eye contact, and smile less after an hour at the reception counter. To change the duties around every hour between telephone, filing, and reception, and to have frequent breaks, will ensure that receptionists retain their welcoming smiles.

Information for patients

New patients need to be made specially welcome, and some practices arrange for them to see their new doctor for a brief session of welcome and explanation of the way the practice works.

Duplicated or printed handouts are particularly welcome. These can take the form of a practice booklet containing all the information, or a series of sheets of paper. Separate sheets are cheaper to produce and easier to update. Each practice will need to follow its own style, but the following information may be included.

Basic information about the practice

1. Description, postal address, and telephone numbers of the practice.
2. Names of doctors, receptionists, and other staff, practice nurses, health visitors, and district nurses.
3. Surgery times, and times for contacting various individuals by telephone (e.g. health visitors).
4. How to reach a doctor in an emergency or out of hours.

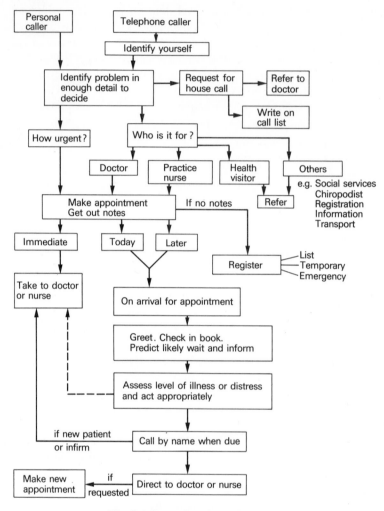

Fig. 8.1. Reception procedures.

Information about practice policies and health education

New patients are particularly impressed by the doctors describing their policies, and showing their concern for their patients' health by including health education material which they endorse. This has particular force when it has the personal imprint of their doctor, and is not just a printed pamphlet (valuable though they may be). Patients get advance warning that the doctors are not in favour of certain remedies (e.g. slimming or sleeping pills) and that they encourage non-smoking. This may save battles in the consulting room. Repeat prescription procedures may be described, with reasons given for surveillance.

Patient-completed questionnaire

A health questionnaire may be given to each patient with a request to complete it and hand it in. This is useful to the doctor in the absence of any medical records, and may alert him to any risk factors. It may contain an invitation to a check of blood pressure, a cervical smear (if appropriate), and completion of courses of immunization which can be arranged direct with the practice nurse.

To produce all these handouts is laborious, but should be undertaken at practice level if it is to be fully effective. The practice manager can obtain examples from other practices and from the Information Resources Centre, and encourage the partners to set out their policies. She must then have them reproduced clearly (e.g. on an IBM composer or similar typewriter at an agency or printer) and then photocopied or duplicated. The next task is to keep them updated as staff, surgery times, or telephone numbers change. Usually the original can be retained and new information typed in using self-adhesive labels or correction fluid. Staff need to be continually reminded to hand them out, and to maintain stocks.

Appointment systems

Appointment systems are not universal, or always popular with everyone, but they are here to stay. They help the doctor to regularize his hours of work, but only help the patient if they are organized efficiently and sensitively.

Spaces must always be reserved, or made, to allow patients who are acutely ill to see a doctor without delay. The patient must decide on the urgency. If the receptionist cannot fit a patient in, only the doctor can decide to send the patient away unseen. Patients who attend their doctor's surgery during surgery hours (as printed in the medical list) have a right to be seen if their condition warrants it. It is a foolhardy receptionist who overrides the patients' assessment of their own need. It would be no problem if there were enough slots free. A rough check can be done each day before closing the surgery – if half the next day's appointment slots are free, then it is likely that the receptionists will be able to cope. If there are very few free slots trouble lies ahead, and urgent steps must be taken to make room – such as prolonging the time of the session, booking more patients so the doctor has to work faster, or arranging extra sessions. The practice manager may be empowered to make such arrangements, even to the extent of getting in a locum to provide an extra pair of hands, and so keep the system flowing smoothly, without the doctors having to worry.

The level of demand should be recorded and monitored by the practice manager, and the monthly and annual statistics presented at practice meetings. Too much overload makes it difficult for patients to see their own personal doctor. Patients prefer to have a personal doctor, and it leads to greater compliance with therapy, better continuity of care, and more effective health education.

The receptionist has an impossible balancing act to perform between too much control in order to provide an ordered flow of booked patients, and the chaos of responding sensitively to peaks of demand by fitting in many acutely ill patients into a 'fully booked' session.

Particular notice needs to be taken of the needs of: children under one, expectant mothers, the elderly, those without telephones or transport, families who are socially disadvantaged, ethnic minorities, those with language difficulties, and individuals with mental handicap. All these categories of people may have difficulty in coping with an appointment system, and so are deterred from seeing a doctor. Many of the categories are associated with risk factors.

For further information on this important topic, the reader is referred to 'Do appointment systems work?' (Arber and Sawyer 1982) and to the *Receptionists' handbook* (DHSS 1981*b*). No appointment system can be perfect, but good design and regular monitoring of its effectiveness (and who can do this better than patients?) are keys to success. Receptionists must be supported by doctors and the practice manager, and helped to express their difficulties and frustrations at regular meetings. Discussion of those patients whom receptionists find difficult will often reveal those with chronic psychiatric illness such as schizophrenia, or mental handicap.

Telephone procedures

Speaking by telephone introduces the barrier of missing the non-verbal cues to communication which we all find so essential. In addition the imperfections of the telephone system can generate much frustration and fury. Many patients have to ring from call-boxes in which the equipment is faulty and they are distracted by traffic noise. They may be unused to the telephone, hard of hearing, and short of coins. Their normal calm may have been disturbed by anxiety and the need to communicate an urgent message. The receptionist must be aware of all these problems and try to compensate for them by extra competence, which can come by training.

Clear procedures must be developed and written down to assist newly-joined staff. The practice manager must ensure that these procedures are adopted, and must train new staff. In some branch exchanges it is all too easy to switch off the incoming call buzzer so that the receptionist must rely on the flashing light, which is not of much use if she has left the switchboard. The Telecom service will arrange training of switchboard operators and telephonists, and will visit any users who are having difficulties.

Procedures will be needed to help receptionists decide whether to put outside calls through to a doctor during consultations. Being accessible to patients by telephone is an essential part of general practice, so compromise is needed. Some doctors have a regular telephone time which is well publicized; some arrange to call patients back (if possible) after surgery. If that is not possible, or the patient considers the message urgent, then the call should be put through. Consultants ringing GPs about their patients get very angry if they are not put through, or just get a recorded message.

Answering machines are valuable for out-of-hours use, when the surgery line cannot be switched through to the partner on duty. They have disadvantages in that they involve the patient in a second phone call, and the machines do not always function properly. Machines which take a message from the patient can be a source of danger, and should be installed only after careful thought.

Requests for home visits

Whether requests come by telephone, by letter, or by a caller, they are fraught with risk. Receptionists can be very anxious in handling such requests, so clear policies and procedures are needed, and training must be extra thorough. The caller will be doubly anxious about the sick person, and about 'bothering the doctor'. The receptionist must be alert to obtain all the necessary information. This includes

(1) identifying particulars, e.g. full name, address, age;
(2) the nature of the trouble – in the caller's own words;
(3) the degree of urgency as stated by the caller;
(4) name of doctor requested and whether registered, temporary patient, or emergency.

This information must all be written down on a message pad or the call book; the time of the message and the doctor's name should be recorded.

The receptionist's next action depends on practice policies. If so authorized she can tell the caller:

'I will tell Dr Smith and he/she will call as soon as possible – ring again if the patient gets worse' or
'I will put you through to speak to Dr Smith (or Dr Jones)' or
'Have you a telephone number, so that Dr Smith can ring you as soon as he/she returns to the surgery?'

The message pad or call book can then be passed to the doctor concerned, the book ticked when the doctor has accepted the call, and the patient's medical record passed to him.

It must be clearly understood by patients, doctors, and receptionists that the receptionist's task is to take the message and pass it quickly to the doctor. She cannot give medical advice, or decide whether a call is necessary. Her manner, style, and training will ensure that the information is of the highest quality, and the patient is confident that the message has been safely received.

If the caller states the need for a visit is urgent or an emergency, the doctor must be told of this immediately. Procedures must be available to guide the receptionist when an emergency call comes in, and there is no doctor in the centre. Radio-telephones or bleeps are very helpful (see Chapter 15). Other options may be to call an ambulance, or a doctor from another practice.

Further information about home visits and emergency cover is available as under:

Sawyer, L. and Arber, S. (1982). Changes in home visiting and night and weekend cover: the patient's view. *British Medical Journal* **284**, 1531–4.

Gray, D. Pereira (1978). Feeling at home. James MacKenzie Lecture 1977. *Journal of the Royal College of General Practitioners* **28**, 6–17.

Other procedures

The practice manager may find it useful for training purposes to codify the good practices which are expected of a receptionist. These could include such topics as:

1. Not keeping a patient waiting at the hatch without good reason and explanation.

2. Not chatting and laughing in the office within sight and hearing of sick patients.

3. Remaining polite under provocation, and using skill in handling aggressive, disturbed, or drunk patients.

4. Explaining to patients about delay when a doctor has been held up or called out.

5. Coping with patients who persistently arrive late.

6. Coping with bereaved or distressed patients.

7. Calling the next patient when the doctor is free.

8. Dealing with patients with potentially infectious complaints so that they may be isolated and seen quickly.

9. Re-stocking the doctor's consulting room with the help of a check-list.

10. Answering patients' enquiries about other staff (e.g. health visitor or social worker) or other agencies, both statutory and voluntary.

11. Displaying and offering health education material on request.

12. Maintaining registers, for example, of workload, hospital transport ordered, hospital appointments and X-rays requested, patients in hospital, and patients who have died.

LANGUAGE AND CULTURAL DIFFERENCES

Mention has been made of the problems of ethnic minorities, which may arise from language difficulties, cultural barriers (such as being examined by a doctor of the opposite sex), and different attitudes to health and to providers of health care. Receptionists need to understand these problems if they are to take part in the educational process to get round the difficulties. They can be helped by such publications as: *Medical practice in a multicultural society* (1988). by J. H. S. Fuller and P. D. Toon. Heinemann Medical, Oxford.

Interpreters may be obtained through social services, or through liaison officers working with local committees for racial integration (details from local Citizens Advice Bureau).

INFORMATION FOR RECEPTIONISTS

Receptionists are asked many questions by patients, some of which may not be relevant to health care. She is expected to have an answer to them all. She cannot expect to have the sources of information available to the Citizens Advice Bureau (CAB), but at least she should know where information can be obtained. For this purpose she will need typed lists of addresses and telephone numbers of a large number of voluntary and statutory agencies. The practice manager will also need a similar information bank (which is considered in Chapter 11), and will want to ensure that receptionists have the information they require. Health visitors and social workers have similar requirements, so liaison can be helpful. When in doubt the CAB is probably the most valuable single source of information, and rarely fails to provide an answer. Receptionists' time can be saved by having a small handout for patients with the most commonly needed addresses and telephone numbers.

Other aspects of the practice organization are considered in subsequent chapters. The receptionist and the practice manager are heavily involved in most of them.

Further reading for receptionists

Drury, M. (1986). *The medical secretary's handbook.* 5th Edn. Baillière Tindall.

McDougall, I. (1980). *Using the telephone.* The Industrial Society, Freepost, London SW1Y 5BR.

DHSS (1981*b*). *The Receptionists' Handbook.* DHSS, London. Available from Stanmore Leaflets Unit, PO Box 21, Stanmore, HA7 1AY.

Stimson, G. and Stimson, C. (1980). *Health rights handbook. A guide to medical care.* Penguin Books.

Video-Arts (1986). *Telephone behaviour: the power and the perils.* Booklet, video tape and film. Video Arts Ltd (address on p 273).

9 Management of prescribing and prescriptions

Prescribing of certain categories of drugs is limited to registered medical practitioners, who carry the responsibility. They can delegate some of the clerical and administrative work to their staff, but the doctor must always sign the prescription, and is responsible for its accuracy.

This chapter is in four sections on: —

management aspects of prescribing;
drug abuse;
repeat prescription procedures;
information about drugs.

All sections concern doctors and some concern practice managers. Dispensing is not considered here.

MANAGEMENT ASPECTS OF PRESCRIBING

General practitioners in the UK write prescriptions costing about £2000 million per annum, which works out at about £36 per patient per annum. This is 50 per cent more than the cost of the general practitioner service.

The cost of prescriptions is rising each year, though the cost relative to total NHS costs is steady. Prescription charges paid by the patient have risen steeply, but large sections of the population are exempt, so only about one third of prescriptions attract a charge. Though the national drug costs seem high, they are well below those of other countries such as USA, France, and Switzerland, both for prescribed drugs and for drugs bought over the counter.

Monitoring of prescribing

Doctors are very free to prescribe what they think will benefit their patient, both in variety and quantity (though a month's supply at a time is regarded as the maximum which should be prescribed). The cost of each GP's prescribing is monitored for one month of each year, and if this is greatly above the local or national average, his attention will be drawn to this fact. Information to the doctor about the quantity and sort of drugs he is prescribing is becoming available with the computerization of the Prescription Pricing Authority, so it will be possible for doctors to know how their prescribing behaviour differs from that of their partners, or from national norms, or 'standards of good practice'. In spite of this monitoring, there are wide variations in prescribing costs between areas, and between individual doctors. Studies of practice activity analysis have shown that doctors vary by a factor of 5 in their prescribing of psychotropic drugs, antibiotics, and so on, and it is difficult to be sure what is 'good' or 'bad' prescribing. It is helpful for the doctor to know where he stands in relation to his colleagues in prescribing various categories of drug. It is a part of the process of performance review, or self-audit.

Practice prescribing policy

Each doctor and each practice will have its policies, but these are rarely written down. It is impossible to lay down policies from outside, but those listed here may form a basis for discussion:

1. Barbiturate hypnotics and slimming tablets will not be prescribed except in special circumstances.

2. Other hypnotic tablets (e.g. Mogadon (Nitrazepam) etc.) will be prescribed for only two weeks at a time, and reviewed monthly by doctor.

3. Other psychotropic drugs will be reviewed every month by the doctor.

4. Patients prescribed psychotropic drugs or antihistamines will (if appropriate) be warned about the danger of driving and UWG (usual warning given) marked in notes.

5. Symptomatic remedies (e.g. cough mixtures, aspirin, paracetamol, etc.) will not be prescribed if it can be avoided. No cough mixtures to be prescribed for children under one year of age.

6. Strong local steroid ointments and creams will not be prescribed for children or for use on the face except in special circumstances.

7. Elderly patients should not be prescribed more than three preparations concurrently, except in special circumstances.

8. When a yellow warning notice is received from the Committee on Safety of Medicines, all patients receiving that particular drug will be reviewed by the doctor immediately.

9. Approved (generic) names of drugs should be used wherever possible.

Most of these policies (or rules) need to be decided by the doctors, if they can agree, but many have management implications. For example, an immediate review of all patients on a particular drug requires a very efficient record system which few practices possess. However the drug is often linked to a diagnosis, so if the practice has a diagnostic index, all the notes can be found, and a quick survey will show which patients are on the offending drug. Other management implications will be discussed in later sections.

Wider implications of prescribing

So far prescribing has been considered mainly at the practice level. What is the management background to prescribing in the National Health Service, and what are the forces at work to influence doctors? This is a very complex subject, which is dealt with in more detail by Mapes (1980), various publications of the Office of Health Economics (OHE), and Pritchard (1981).

As mentioned previously, the general practitioner has considerable freedom to prescribe, but he is subject to a number of influences which are outlined in Fig. 9.1. Doctors are under some pressure from their patients to prescribe, but they also influence patients to accept a prescription, as one way of terminating the interview – 'a disengaging device' (Mapes 1980).

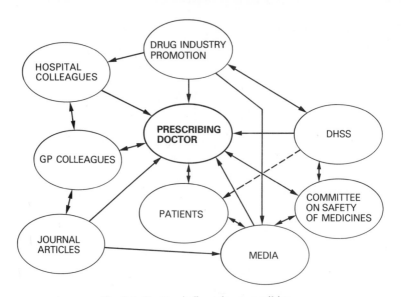

Fig. 9.1. Factors influencing prescribing.

Not all prescriptions are taken to the pharmacist, nor are all medicines collected. When collected, the medicines may be hoarded or discarded. This is more likely to happen when the pressure to prescribe comes from the doctor, but the patient has other aims, e.g. just a talk to relieve anxiety, or a certificate. It has also been shown that 'compliance' with medicine-taking is better when the practice operates a personal-doctor system (see Chapter 8).

The doctor is under strong influence from pharmaceutical firms to prescribe their branded products. Their expensive promotion is effective. Drug firms may spend many millions of pounds on developing a new drug, so it is reasonable that they should recoup their development costs, or innovation would cease. It is important to distinguish between new products which really provide better treatment (e.g. cimetidine, which has reduced costs spent on surgical treatment), and those elegant cough medicines or skin creams which have little proven value. It is important for pharmaceutical firms to market a new drug quickly, before it is imitated, or patents expire; whereas slower introduction would allow closer monitoring of adverse reactions. The Committee on Safety of Medicines (CSM) marks certain new products in *MIMS* where special alertness to side effects, and special reporting to the CSM is advised by yellow card.

Prescribing doctors are flooded with information from drug firms, but most general practitioners behave critically, and do not believe all they are told. They have a natural distrust of promotion, and need a new drug to be 'legitimized', by its prescribing by hospital consultants or colleagues. Publications such as *Drug and therapeutics bulletin* provide criticism of unfounded claims, and generally adopt a cautious line. The DHSS looks at costs, and provides some monitoring through its Regional Medical Service. There is less DHSS monitoring of hospital doctors, but some hospitals have an active monitoring and educational approach in which general practice is included.

Financial implications

When we turn attention to money, we detect an inherently unstable pattern (see Fig. 9.2). The prescribing doctor is much more strongly influenced by the drug firm than by the DHSS, and has little or no incentive to prescribe economically. The DHSS (through the FPC or health board) automatically picks up the bill, and has virtually no budgetary or financial control, as would be normal in any other industrial setting. One would expect drug costs to escalate, and indeed they have done so; it is surprising that they have not gone completely wild. Restraint by doctors and the industry is part of the reason, and the DHSS has agreements with the industry on price levels and promotion expenditure.

The message for those who plan and administer health care is clear. Here is a substantial area of expenditure where budgetary control does not exist, and

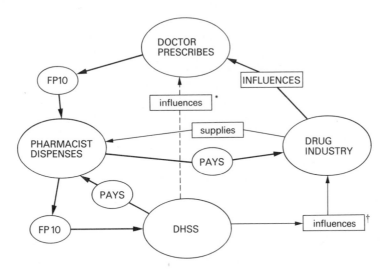

Fig. 9.2. The prescribing 'money go round'. **Prescriber's journal.* Annual costs. †Price agreement.

whose effectiveness is in serious doubt. It is in the interest of general practitioners to monitor the effectiveness of their prescribing and ask if the money is well spent – or could it be better spent in other areas of primary health care which are at present starved of funds? An 'open-ended' drug budget is an anachronism in times of financial stringency, and general practitioners are in danger of losing the privilege if they do not put their house in order.

Monitoring the effectiveness of prescribing is a major task which is only touched upon in this chapter. Further information can be sought from Marsh (1981) who describes a safe and economical prescribing routine using a 'minicopoea', and Tulloch (1981) who reviews repeat prescribing in elderly patients.

The role of the drug firm representative

Figure 9.1 indicates the strong influence of the drug industry on prescribing in general practice. Though advertising and sponsorship play their part, the major influence on the doctor's prescribing is the drug firm representative. This perhaps accounts for their numbers and enthusiasm. It is not unusual for three representatives to arrive in one morning and expect to see the doctor. The practice manager has an important mediating role in protecting the doctor's time yet ensuring that he obtains the information he wants. The receptionist, too, needs support if she has to turn away keen (and persuasive) representatives. Once again a practice policy, or failing that a policy for each doctor, is needed about which firm's representatives will be seen, for how long, at what intervals, and how many in a week.

Some practices have a policy of not seeing drug firm representatives at all. Once the decision is known, the drug firms respect it, and life is made easier for the receptionists, and probably for the doctor also. Anxieties among doctors that they will miss out on valuable information are probably unfounded, as general practitioners are overloaded with information about drugs. The loss of all the diaries, notepads, and gimmicky gifts which tend to clutter up the doctor's desk, has to be borne with fortitude. Another loss is the company of the drug representatives, chosen for their charm and personality, which many doctors find a pleasant diversion after a busy surgery.

DRUG ABUSE

Doctors are under pressure to prescribe controlled drugs (drugs listed in the Misuse of Drugs Act 1971) from addicts, or from those who wish to sell them on the black market for cash. This can involve the doctor in severe penalties if he complies with their requests. Details of the legislation can be found in the *British National Formulary*.

Similar problems can arise with temporary residents who request prescriptions for psychotropic drugs like sleeping tablets, tranquillizers, or slimming tablets. They usually tell a very convincing story. It is a wise precaution to telephone their registered general practitioner first, and in cases of doubt to telephone the FPC or Health Board, who keep a register of such people. Practices usually receive circulars about persistent drug abusers, and it is helpful if the practice manager keeps the file up-to-date and accessible to doctors and receptionists. Any doubtful temporary resident can quickly be checked against the file, and the doctor alerted. Another common abuse of health care is for patients to steal FP10s or copies of *MIMS* which have a high black market value, so their security should be under constant review.

REPEAT PRESCRIPTION PROCEDURES

General practitioners are often criticized for the amount of repeat prescribing which they do – sometimes amounting to 50 per cent of the total prescriptions. Some of the criticism arises from inadequate procedures for review, so that people go on taking drugs unnecessarily. However, the work of Balint *et al.* (1970) threw doubt on the whole question of repeat prescribing: 'The repeat prescription is a diagnosis that something has gone wrong in the doctor–patient relationship'. 'The patient accepts the drug as a symbol of something he badly needs'. The doctor colludes guiltily, knowing that there is little pharmacological justification for his prescribing, but it is the easy way out.

How can a proper balance be struck between inappropriate and unsupervised prescribing or over-prescribing and a convenient service for patients who properly need regular treatment? How can administrative staff play a role without having to take responsibility for medical decisions?

Before describing procedures of repeat prescriptions, let us consider who does it and where. Unless the practice has a dispenser, probably a senior receptionist will write the repeat prescriptions for the doctor to sign. She will need training in correct prescription writing, and perhaps a friendly local pharmacist would help her. Cruickshank's book *The pocket prescriber, and guide to prescription writing* (Livingstone £1.25) might be helpful.

Prescribing is such an important task that the work-station needs some thought. A separate desk for writing prescriptions is an advantage; it can be used by the staff for writing them, and by the doctors for signing. it is a good place to collect all the possible sources of information about prescribing, which are considered in the next section. An office desk with lockable drawers for the FP10s (which must be kept under lock and key) and a filing drawer will suffice. There should be a bookshelf within reach, and a pin-board for notices. A telephone extension is an advantage. Ready access to patients' medical records is essential.

Repeat prescribing—the practice manager's role

Some patients are on a regular drug regime which means that they can request repeat prescriptions without seeing the doctor every time. This will be particularly useful for the chronically sick patient. The patient will normally be given the prescription on a monthly basis and be seen by the doctor at three-monthly intervals, perhaps longer, perhaps less, depending on the patient's need. This seems a sensible arrangement, but the repeat prescription service remains a problem area, in which mistakes may have serious consequences. The doctor must sign the prescription, and is responsible for its accuracy and appropriateness. The patient must not get the impression that the receptionist decides what drugs are prescribed, nor that the drugs can be obtained on demand, like shopping at a supermarket.

The doctor will expect the receptionist to help him by:

1. Taking note and recording the patient's request, (by letter, personal call, or by telephone).

2. Handling the clerical aspects of the request.

3. Ensuring the doctor deals with the request.

4. Ensuring the patient gets his prescription form.

5. Teaching the patient how to obtain the best service.

The receptionist must have crystal-clear instructions and never be placed in the position of making a medical decision.

There are many ways of running an effective repeat prescription service. So how will the practice manager help to set up a system which best suits the patients and the practice? She may want to ask some questions. For example:

1. Can the information of drug requirements be extracted easily from the NHS record card? Is it absolutely clear what drugs the patient is receiving?

2. Are drug sensitivities clearly marked? (Preferably boldly in red.)

3. Having agreed that the drug information must be clearly and quickly identified, does the practice wish:

(a) to continue to use its present form of recording?

(b) to introduce a special drug record card/sheet to be kept in the notes, which will be separate from all other entries?

(c) to introduce a special card/sheet for repeat prescribing only?

4. What are the advantages to the patient and to the practice of giving the patient a repeat prescription card?

5. Will there be a standard policy for review of repeat prescriptions? For example, will the patient be asked to make an appointment with the doctor after three months? How will the doctor indicate any change to the standard routine?

6. How much of the prescription form does the general practitioner envisage the receptionist being able to complete? If she is to write the complete prescription, has she been suitably trained? Is she aware of the regulations about controlled drugs?

7. Are there clear rules about preventing forgery, (e.g. drawing of an oblique line below the last prescription, and ringing the quantity to be dispensed), and about controlled drugs?

8. Is the service to be provided 'while you wait', or the next day?

9. Will there be age restrictions on accepting requests and giving out prescriptions (e.g. aged 16 or over)?

10. Is there a clear policy to ensure the safety of blank prescription forms?

11. What procedures will there be to avoid confusion of names, so that the patient is given the right prescription?

12. Are the policies and procedures written down and regularly updated?

What will the patient need to know?

The doctor is responsible for issuing the initial prescription, and for explaining to the patient what the preparation is, what it is aimed to do, and possible side effects. The doctor will no doubt explain in the first instance, but will the patient remember?

The receptionist may be the most appropriate person to discuss with the patient how to make the most of the repeat prescription service. The patient will possibly feel that the doctor is far too busy to spell out the enormously long name of the new drug. The patient may well find difficulty in pronouncing it, let alone spelling it! The receptionist will be able to suggest appropriate times to telephone with requests, whether the practice will accept written requests, or whether arrangements can be made to post prescriptions to infirm or house-bound patients. The receptionist will be able to explain the need for a 'next day' service and that the patient will be reminded in perhaps three months time to make an appointment to see the doctor. A typed slip to explain why this is necessary may save many phone calls from angry patients.

The repeat prescription service is not only to save doctors' time but also to suit the needs of patients. Unreasonable requests must be resisted in the interests of the patient, as well as the public purse. The library of the Royal College of General Practitioners and the Information Resources Centre can offer much assistance on repeat prescription services and systems. Drury's paper on repeat prescribing† should be read for further information.

INFORMATION ABOUT PRESCRIBING

New and powerful drugs are available which produce profound physiological changes in the body. It is no wonder that side effects are becoming an increasing problem. It is estimated that drug-induced disease accounts for between 3 and 5 per cent of hospital admissions. Some drugs are incompatible with each other, or affect each others action in a way that the doctor must be aware of. The number and range of incompatibilities is so great that it is difficult to remember them all, and mistakes often occur.

All these factors call for a good information system about drugs which needs to be:

up-to-date;
comprehensive;

†Drury, V. W. M. (1982). Repeat prescribing – a review. *Journal of the Royal College of General Practitioners.* **32**, 42–5.

reliable;
readily accessible;
clearly understood.

Books and periodicals

The British national formulary (BNF). This is regularly updated, and it should be the book of first reference, as its index contains approved names and proprietary names. It also gives the prescriber the opportunity to prescribe good old-fashioned non-proprietary remedies which may be just as effective, and will certainly be cheaper than proprietary drugs. The number of occasions when it is necessary to prescribe a drug not in the *BNF* should be very few. By grouping preparations logically it is easier to compare alternatives, as well as price bands.

The *BNF* is published jointly by the British Medical Association and the Pharmaceutical Society of Great Britain, and is issued free to NHS doctors, but may also be purchased from the publishers.

Monthly index of medical specialties (MIMS). This indispensable reference book has the advantage of being up-to-date, and having several useful sections such as a cross-index of approved and proprietary names, and a list of dressings and appliances and borderline substances. It contains details of about 2000 drugs. Thirty-six drugs are thought adequate for over 80 per cent of prescriptions (Marsh 1981).

The data sheet compendium. This is published annually by the Association of the British Pharmaceutical Industry. It summarizes the data sheets (see below), and so is a convenient collection of information. The order of entries is at first confusing, as they are grouped under the various manufacturers, and not all drug firms contribute. It is issued free to NHS principals.

Safer prescribing, 2nd Edn, by Beeley, L. (1979). Blackwell Scientific Publications, £1.75. A valuable pocket guide to drug interactions and prescribing problems.

Textbooks on adverse drug reactions. e.g. those by Davies, D. M. 2nd Edn. Oxford University Press, £30 (or available through Medicine Book Club); or Wade, O. L. 2nd Edn. Heinemann, £3.20.

Textbooks of Pharmacology and Therapeutics. There is a wide choice, and the following are recommended:
Dilling, W. J. (1979). *Clinical pharmacology,* 24th Edn. Baillière, £9.75.
Laurence, D. R. (1980). *Clinical pharmacology,* 5th Edn. Churchill Livingstone, £11.00.
Turner, P. and Richens, A. (1978). *Clinical pharmacology* 3rd Edn. Churchill Livingstone, £3.50.

Drug and therapeutics bulletin. This is a most valuable critical guide to treatment. Published fortnightly by the Consumers' Association. Issued free to NHS GPs. Box files and index available.

Prescribers journal. Issued quarterly by the DHSS to all NHS doctors. Contains useful articles about drugs and treatment.

A Pharmacopeia, such as Martindale, *The extra pharmacopeia* is perhaps a luxury for non-dispensing practice.

Other sources of information

Information on file

Files should be kept on information about:

(1) vaccines and immunization;

(2) yellow warning notices from the Committee on Safety of Medicine;

(3) drug interactions – also available as posters and plastic dials;

(4) data sheets. It is only necessary to keep those published since the last data sheet compendium and those not included;

(5) file of notices from FPC about people who use assumed names to obtain drugs.

Information on pin-board

This should include:

(1) telephone numbers of outside sources of information;

(2) drug interaction poster.

Outside sources of information

Most queries can be answered from the references quoted above, but it is essential to have easy access to outside sources of information.

The local pharmacist may be the first source of advice, or alternatively the district hospital pharmacist will usually be pleased to help with GPs queries. For more medical questions the consultant clinical pharmacologist offers an advisory service, usually at regional level.

For advice about poisoning, there are five National Poisons Information Service Centres. Their telephone numbers are as follows:

Belfast	0232 240503 ext. 2140	Edinburgh	031 229 2477 ext. 2233
Birmingham	021 554 3801 ext. 4109	London	01 635 9191
Cardiff	0222 569200	Newcastle	091 232 1525 or 5131
Dublin	0001 74 5588		

Medical information departments of pharmaceutical firms are very helpful. Telephone numbers are given in *MIMS*.

Advice about immunization, particularly that for travellers may be obtained from:

The Institute of Tropical Hygiene, tel. 01 636 8636, ext. 212.

Medical Information Department, Wellcome Foundation, tel. 0270 583151.

DHSS International Division, tel. 01 407 5522, ext. 6711.

The local community physician, or infectious diseases consultant.

Prestel (see below).

Computer-based drug information, such as that operated by Prestel, is the ideal solution for the future, and some local systems are already in operation.

Access may be obtained by a telephone line with a visual display unit. Prestel are developing a national service on these lines. It might not be economical to have a set solely for drug information, but it could be part of a practice computer installation (see Chapter 12).

One way of cutting down on prescribing is by keeping people well and preventing illness! This is considered in the next chapter.

10 Prevention in primary health care

The successes of medicine in the past 100 years have been mostly in the field of prevention. Examples are the eradication of smallpox; immunization against diphtheria, poliomyelitis, tuberculosis, and measles; and the prevention of malaria. Against this can be set the epidemic of diseases associated with people's life-style and behaviour, many of which should be preventable. Examples are coronary thrombosis, lung cancer, bronchitis, sexually transmitted disease, alcoholism, and road accidents. There is another group of diseases in which early detection and treatment can reduce the danger – for example, high blood pressure and cancer of the uterine cervix (neck of the womb).

There are thus three kinds of approach:

1. To eradicate or reduce disease by improvements in hygiene and by immunization.

2. To help people to alter their behaviour where this may lead to ill-health: 'health promotion'.

3. By searching out the early signs of certain diseases where this has been shown to be worthwhile: 'case-finding' or 'screening'. †

Many of the decisions about promoting health have to be taken at national level – concerning, for example, the advertising of cigarettes, and seat-belt legislation. But much can be done at general-practice level in helping patients to think ahead, and to avoid unpleasant consequences. To do so involves some change in the style of general practice: from waiting until things go wrong then trying to put them right, to programmes of immunization, education, or case-finding which can be thought of as 'anticipatory care'. Doctors need to change their attitudes and so do patients if an improvement in health is to be achieved. Different methods of working may be needed, in which management support is a key factor.

What preventive measures are worth taking in general practice, and what are the management implications? A list of suggested measures is given in Table 10.1. Each practice must make its own list in the light of the best advice available at the time, and decide on priorities.

---

†There is some ambiguity in the terms 'case-finding' and 'screening'. Strictly the former is the detection of people who have symptoms which they have not reported, whereas the latter is the detection of disease before symptoms have appeared.

Table 10.1. *Preventive measures worth taking in general practice*

Group at risk	Measures to be considered
(i) Pre-conception	Ensuring rubella immunity, good nutritional status, and knowledge of care in early pregnancy
(ii) Antenatal	Regular attendance at antenatal clinic. α-feto-protein test, etc.
(iii) Postnatal	Check physical status, psychological state, e.g. depression, and bonding of mother and child
(iv) First year of life	Check for congenital dislocation of hip, phenylketonuria, etc. Immunize against diphtheria, pertussis, tetanus, and poliomyelitis. Check hearing, and vision. At risk register
(v) Age one to five	Give measles vaccination, and diphtheria/tetanus, poliomyelitis boosters. Check hearing and vision. Accident risks
(vi) School age	Immunize against rubella, tuberculosis, and diphtheria/tetanus/polio. Check hearing and vision. Health promotion – non-smoking, exercise, weight control, interpersonal relationships
(vii) Adult	Health promotion – non-smoking, exercise, weight control. Check blood pressure. Psychiatric disorders, including bereavement counselling. Care of diabetes, and chronic diseases. Females – contraception, cervical screening, (?) breast examination.
(viii) Elderly	Screening for preventable or treatable disability, and socio-medical problems. Appropriateness of prescribing

IMPLICATIONS FOR MANAGEMENT

Much will depend on the doctors' policies and the way they view their work (see Chapters 4 and 7). However, those doctors who do not have the enthusiasm to initiate preventive work in the practice, may be prepared to let it happen if the process is painless. This is where good management can help to support a preventive approach, so that it is easy for both doctors and patients to accept it. Who are the people involved in prevention?

Key role of health visitor

Prevention, health promotion, and education are all part of the health visitor's job and training. Her advice and co-operation must be sought at an early stage. For prevention to be effective, there must be good teamwork (see Chapter 6). The health visitor has good links with the resources of the health-education unit of the District Health Authority.

Other team members

A practice policy of achieving as much prevention of illness as resources allow will involve all members of the team; some preventive procedures (outlined later) will concern them. They all have an opportunity to set an example in healthy living. In some practices none of the doctors nor staff smoke, and some run their own keep-fit, slimming, and relaxation classes.

The community physician

Prevention, epidemiology, and planning are all within the remit of the community medicine specialist based at district (DMO). As well as providing expertise, he is able to call on funds for specific projects, and monitor the outcome of preventive programmes. Rather than wait for the DMO to call, it might be an idea to invite him to the practice to discuss strategies for prevention, and ways of implementing them.

The general practitioner

Several studies have shown that the general practitioner in the consultation has an exceptional opportunity to influence his patient's behaviour. The opportunity may arise from the topic of the consultation (e.g. patient with a cough being advised to stop smoking), or the doctor may introduce the subject. Patients resent this less than one expects, so long as the advice is given sensitively and with due regard to their personal beliefs about health and the causes and risks of ill health (King 1983). Advice about health behaviour is more likely to be acceptable from a personal doctor who is known and trusted (see Chapter 8). Above all the general practitioner has a chance to lead by his example of healthy living.

The patient

Behavioural change primarily involves the patient whose health it is, so each patient's responsibility should be encouraged. Self-help groups (see later) and patient participation (see Chapter 6) are potent instruments of health education.

Having outlined the cast, we can now consider what action is needed for prevention of specific diseases, or for promotion of health. It will be possible to take only some examples from the list in Table 10.1 for detailed study, but the general principles of management described in this book should be applicable. (See in particular objectives in Chapter 7 and planning in Chapter 17.) Let us now see where the practice manager fits in to the picture and what role she can play.

WHAT CAN THE PRACTICE MANAGER DO?

Pre-conception

Antenatal care must start before conception, but this group of women is very hard to identify as so many pregnancies are unplanned. Screening for rubella immunity can be undertaken for all young women on the contraceptive pill, by incorporating it in the clerical procedures for pill-checks (see later).

Current advice about pre-conception nutrition, tablet and alcohol taking, early antenatal attendance, etc. needs to be widely available to women of child-bearing age – perhaps posters and simple handouts could be devised by the health visitor and the health education unit.

Antenatal

Antenatal care needs to be sensitive to the individual feelings of each pregnant woman, so too much regimentation or coercion may be counter-productive. On the other hand, the system needs to be 100 per cent fail-safe.

As soon as pregnancy is confirmed the patient must be encouraged to see the doctor – perhaps at an ordinary surgery if she is not keen to identify herself at the clinic. A code-mark for pregnant women attending is helpful, so that non-attendance is notified immediately to the doctor or midwife, and appropriate action taken. After one default, the next appointment can be underlined in red, so that a second non-attendance results in a request for the midwife to visit at home. Similarly in the antenatal clinic, the system needs to be designed so that no one misses key times for check-ups if humanly possible.

For those patients having shared home and hospital care there is a particular risk of the hospital and general practitioner thinking that the other is doing the checks. Meticulous attention to co-operation cards, and liaison with hospital appointment clerks, will obviate this slip-up. A check-list on the co-operation card for the various time-sensitive procedures like α-feto-protein testing can be helpful, so that a non-event is detected immediately. Poorer sections of the community are at particular risk, so special attention is needed to ensure that they do not miss out.

Postnatal

The practice manager is concerned with efficient documentation, including claims for maternity services, which are normally completed and sent off at the postnatal visit. Mothers with older children find it particularly difficult to attend, as do mothers who are depressed, or those with transport difficulties. The postnatal visit is an opportunity to detect whether a mother is depressed, or when their is a disturbance of mother–child bonding, both of which may need treatment.

First year of life

Infants under one year of age are at particular risk from infections, and it is a time of great anxiety for mothers. Close liaison with the health visitor about ill babies or those at risk is essential. Some babies may not be registered with the practice; some families may have moved and the health visitor does not have the address. Close attention to detail, and efficient reception and clerical procedures with this age group in mind will help.

A practice in Birmingham (Pike 1980) issues a booklet and a priority card to mothers of all children under one, which allows the child to be seen without an appointment and without delay. It has worked well.

A number of health checks need to be carried out in infancy and it is not enough to assume that they have been done at the Child Health Clinic. Attendance at clinics is not 100 per cent, and the non-attenders tend to be those in greatest need (social class V). Again, close liaison with the health visitor, and a check of names against the practice age–sex register is useful.

Immunization is a complex administrative problem, requiring children to attend on four occasions in the first 13 months at certain ages and intervals. The appointments must be convenient for the mother, and the child must be well. Failed appointments must be followed up. With good procedures it is possible to achieve 100 per cent immunization (apart from a few refusals). Most practitioners have the benefit of a computerized recall system run by the health authority. It is only as good as the data it receives, so new arrivals, changes of address, etc. must be fed in. An equally efficient manual system is described in Appendix A.

Age one to five

Health checks and immunization appointments are needed in this age group also. Accidents are a particular hazard to these children, so a programme of health education co-ordinated by the health visitor is appropriate. The practice manager's help will be needed in devising procedures, and in making sure that things turn out as planned.

School age

Immunization against rubella (german measles), tuberculosis, and diphtheria, tetanus and polio boosters are usually advised for school children. If a check is made against the practice age–sex register of children immunized against rubella at school, it may be found that only half the children were immunized, and no follow up carried out. The practice manager can institute such a check, or alternatively flag the notes of all the children aged 11 to ensure that their rubella immunity is questioned at the next attendance. Those who miss the injection at school can be immunized at the surgery and a fee claimed.

Many of the habits which affect health in later life develop at school, so health promotion must start at school. Many education authorities do not give health education a high priority, and tend to leave it to the health education service, the school nursing service, or, where this is lacking, to health visitors. Unless education for health is an integral part of education for living, then it will be regarded as an optional special subject. General practitioners can use their authority in the community to influence these issues, and may find it worthwhile, with the health visitors, to take part in the health education of pupils (and teachers) in school.

Adults

There are so many facets of health promotion and case-finding or screening for disease in adult life, that we must be selective. What measures have been shown to be effective, and what are the priorities?

Smoking is the major hazard to health today, causing 200 deaths a day, and being the major risk factor in lung cancer, bronchitis, and coronary thrombosis, as well as being a contributory factor in many other cancers. One smoker in four dies of a smoking-related disease, and a large proportion of NHS resources – including the time of general practitioners is taken up with the care of these sufferers.

Prevention of arterial disease

Myocardial infarcts (coronary thrombosis, or heart attacks), strokes, hypertension (high blood pressure), and obstruction of leg arteries are manifestations of arterial disease. It is thought that half the strokes, and one quarter of myocardial infarcts under age 70, are preventable. The latter causes about half the deaths of people aged 45–65 (RCGP 1981c).

The major risk factors in myocardial infarction are:

smoking;
obesity;
hypertension;
lack of exercise;
diabetes;
hereditary.

Many of these factors react with one another (see Fig. 10.1) and have different effects in different categories of arterial disease. Smoking, in addition to being a major risk factor in myocardial infarction, and obstruction of leg arteries, is also the major cause of lung cancer, bronchitis, and emphysema, and is an important factor in cancer of the mouth, larynx, oesophagus, and bladder. It is thought to be responsible for about one third of all cancer deaths (Doll and Peto 1981). Dietary fibre may protect against arterial disease and cancer of the bowel, as well as having other beneficial effects.

Rather than launch a number of programmes for preventing specific diseases, it might be simpler – in view of the overlapping effect of several risk factors – to devise a programme for healthy living which people can be helped to follow. This would have the following elements:

(1) give up smoking
(2) keep body weight within reasonable limits;
(3) limit intake of animal fat;
(4) take adequate fibre in diet;
(5) take adequate daily exercise;
(6) detect and treat arterial hypertension;
(7) detect and treat diabetes.

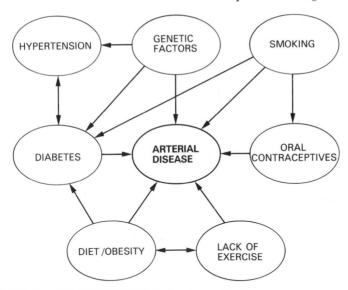

Fig. 10.1. Risk factors in arterial disease.

Other areas in which preventive medicine might well be applied to adults are:

(1) reduction of prescribing of potentially toxic drugs;
(2) limitation of alcohol abuse;
(3) prevention or early treatment of certain psychiatric disorders (RCGP 1981d);
(4) a well supervised family-planning service (RCGP 1981e);
(5) in females, a cervical screening service, and possibly breast screening.

We have already opened up a large area of activity which would be very difficult to implement in general practice. For further details the reader is referred to Fowler and Gray (1982) or the reports from the Royal College of General Practitioners (RCGP 1981b–e).

As examples of the way in which a practice manager can help in the implementation of preventive programmes in adults, the following have been selected;

give up smoking;
detection and treatment of hypertension;
cervical screening.

'Give up smoking'

Advice from general practitioners to their patients to give up smoking has been shown to be followed in about 5 per cent of cases (Russell *et al.* 1979). If all general practitioners gave anti-smoking advice, backed up by a leaflet and a promise of follow up, it would produce the same effect as 10000 special anti-smoking clinics.

The steps in a drive to reduce smoking in the practice population could be as follows:

1. Record the smoking habits of all adult patients in the notes at their next attendance. Coloured labels (green for non-smokers, fluorescent orange or red for smokers) can be stuck in the margin of the notes. In the case of smokers, the number or amount smoked can be written on the label. Anyone handling the notes in the presence of the patient could do this, i.e. receptionist, practice nurse, or doctor.

2. Doctor draws the attention of all patients to the risks of smoking, particularly those with arterial disease or other risk factors.

3. Doctor chooses a suitable moment to recommend patient strongly to give up smoking.

4. At the same time, hand patient a booklet such as *Give up smoking* or *So you want to stop smoking.* †

5. Put patient in touch with self help groups in area – a typed address slip is helpful.

6. Ask about smoking at follow-up visits, and record progress in notes.

7. Set an example in non-smoking.

8. Display suitable posters and non-smoking stickers in waiting room.

9. Pay particular attention to smoking in pregnancy.

The practice manager can help by having a practice policy defined and agreed. A supply of sticky labels, pamphlets, and address slips should be available at all sites where they might be needed. Doctors' desk and car stocks will need to be checked. Evaluation of the success of the project would need a special study, i.e. check notes daily before filing to count how many green labels have been affixed, where previously there was a red one, and record weekly total of successes (and backsliders).

Detection and treatment of hypertension

It is generally agreed that the numbers of deaths from arterial disease can be reduced by treating all people with a diastolic‡ blood pressure of 105 mmHg and over, with the aim of bringing it down to about 80 mmHg. Whether to treat people with a diastolic blood pressure between 90 and 104 mmHg has been in doubt, but recent studies have shown that death rates can be reduced markedly by treatment. Against this must be set the risk of drug side effects, and a threefold increase in workload for hypertension. Drug costs will be high, but the improvement in health should more than justify such a policy.

When planning the programme, certain decisions will have to be taken:

†Obtainable free from local health education unit or Health Education Authority, 78 New Oxford Street, London WC1A 1AH.

‡Blood comes from the heart into the arteries in a wave, whose pressure at the peak of the wave is called 'systolic' and in the trough 'diastolic'.

1. 'Case-finding' of people who present themselves at the surgery, or total population screening. †

2. Age range to be covered, e.g. 30–64 initially, extending to 20–69 if programme goes well.

3. Limits of blood pressure – the three-box system (Hart 1980) (see Table 10.2).

4. Additional staff needed, cost, and so on.

5. Staff training and motivation.

6. Resources needed – cash, stationery, etc.

7. When to start.

8. When to evaluate.

Table 10.2 *The 'three-box system' for blood pressure screening*

	Age under 40	Age 40–64
For treatment	Over 165/100	Over 180/105
For observation after one year	140/85 to 164/99	155/90 to 179/104
For re-check after five years	Less than 140/85	Less than 155/90

A flow chart (Fig. 10.2) illustrates the procedures for a case-finding plan for a practice population of 10 000. In screening those aged 20–65 one would expect to find 308 hypertensives and 280 borderline cases. An operational check list is included as Appendix B.

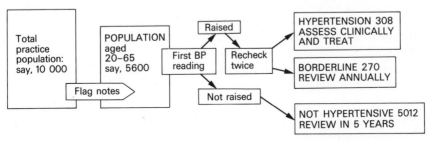

Fig. 10.2. Flow chart of hypertension case finding. (Based on Hart (1980) Appendix I.)

Cervical screening

Screening of women aged 35–64 for cancer of the uterine cervix (neck of the womb) has been shown to be effective, and is recommended government policy.

† Four out of every five registered patients consult their doctors each year, so that adequate case-finding can be achieved by catching people who present themselves. A fuller screening programme based on the practice list is more difficult and expensive. For those with a computerized age–sex register, it is relatively simple.

To further this aim, general practitioners are currently paid £5.70 (1984) for every test completed. The tests can be carried out by the doctor, or by a suitably trained practice nurse. The details will vary according to practice circumstances. For a draft operational plan see Appendix C.

Contraception

This is an important area of preventive medicine. The management of a recall system is described in Appendices A, B, and C. For further reading see Bull (1982) and RCGP (1981e).

The elderly

Many of the preventive measures for adults apply equally to the elderly who are not, after all, a separate species, but a few years older. However, certain disabilities can have a serious impact on independence in later life, so preventive work may be worthwhile. This is often called 'Geriatric Screening' and is aimed to detect treatable physical and social conditions which may limit the quality of life, as well as putting a strain on services.

The numbers of the elderly in the population are likely to increase considerably in the next 20 years. However, those retiring now are in much better health than those who retired 25 years ago, and who may be in residential care, so the outlook is not as black as the figures suggest.

The evidence for geriatric screening being effective is difficult to assess, but those who have tried it usually think it worthwhile. Elderly people are reluctant to seek medical help, and unmet need is common. This issue is treated at greater length in Wilcock *et al.* (1982). Sample procedures and proforma for a geriatric survey follow (see Appendix D). Such a survey depends on a high level of co-operation from the Health Visitor and District Nurse. The practice manager's liaison and co-ordinating skills will be fully taxed in keeping such a complicated process going.

Prevention of accidents and hypothermia in the elderly are a high priority, and reference should be made to Wilcock *et al.* (1982).

SELF-HELP GROUPS IN GENERAL PRACTICE

Groups run mainly by patients for mutual benefit operate at various levels. At the practice or local level, it is common to have groups for slimming, keep fit, or giving up smoking based on the practice. Many other kinds of group can flourish as described by Williamson and Danaher (1977). Some groups operate locally with the focus on a specific disease or disability (e.g asthma, psoriasis, alcoholism, diabetes). Many of these groups have powerful and efficient national organizations which are of great benefit to individual patients and act as a national pressure-group. There are over 200 of these, and they are usually listed in a directory held at the local Citizen's Advice Bureau, or the Council for

Voluntary Organizations. Pull-out supplements in papers like *Pulse* and *General Practitioner* are useful and should be filed.

Some groups are less formally organized, e.g. those aiming to help people suffering from stress or agoraphobia, or needing some sort of support, for example, after cot-death or bereavement. They may have difficulty in finding somewhere to meet, and lack the administrative framework needed to run a small organization. A helping hand from the practice may ensure the survival of these very useful groups. Such support should be unobtrusive, with as little professional dominance as possible, or the group will disappear.

HEALTH EDUCATION

Ideas are changing about the most effective ways of informing people about health issues, and encouraging them to change their behaviour in the direction of healthy living.

Media campaigns, posters, harangues, or lectures are relatively ineffective, because they do not relate to the beliefs that individuals hold about health, or to the risks that people perceive in their daily living. This means that health education must be a two-way process, with the educator listening to the learner. Perhaps this is why the GP's advice to give up smoking is so effective. The transaction is 'one-to-one', and the doctor may be aware of the patient's beliefs, and the risk he attaches to smoking.

Community-based health education is more likely to succeed than class-room learning. Fellow members of the community may be more acceptable as teachers than professionals, so self-help groups may be more effective than lectures from doctors. An interesting compromise has been tried experimentally in Bristol, where all the practice population at risk for certain illnesses were given a personal invitation to attend a session organized by the practice patients' association. About one quarter of those at risk attended, and nearly all found it to be helpful.

The health visitor will be in touch with community-based health education. The practice manager can ensure that the whole team knows what is going on and reinforce the message. Many options for prevention are open in general practice, (see Fowler and Gray 1982, RCGP 1981b, and Pike 1982). The practice manager can help the team to study the options and decide between them. Once the decision is made she can start on the very major management task which preventive medicine entails.

11 Medical records and information

WHY KEEP RECORDS?

The format of general practitioners' medical records has been virtually unchanged since 1912. Only lately have A4 size (30×21 cm)† records been introduced to a few fortunate practices. The records are technically 'the property of the minister', but they are treated confidentially by lay clerks. Although NHS doctors are supposed, by statute, to keep records, 'in such a form as the Minister may from time to time determine', in practice they record what they think fit, and this varies widely.

Records are kept in general practice for a number of different reasons, by doctors, nurses, and administrative staff. Can we first ask ourselves why?

Medical records have six main functions, listed below:

A permanent record of significant events

In this respect it is an unique health record, as it should be a continuing record of health and illness from birth to death. It does not always achieve this aim, partly because significant events are not always recorded in the right person's notes, and partly because records get lost, and the new ones which are constructed contain no past data. Even when the significant events in a record are summarized, the accuracy is not very high.

A medico-legal record

This aspect is of considerable importance, should a complaint or legal action arise. Negative information may be just as important as positive, such as 'X-ray normal'.

A way of communicating with colleagues and other team members

The single-handed doctor of bygone days only needed to remind himself. Now with partners, deputies, and teams it is important that all should be aware of the main facts such as past and present diagnoses, current treatment, and any allergies or warnings.

A file for hospital and laboratory reports and letters

This information needs to be accessible, or it is useless. A4 files are much better in this respect, but are a temptation to file rather than throw away useless or duplicated information.

† This is the paper size. The file cover is about 31 × 24cm.

An aide memoire

It is important that a patient's personal doctor can remind himself what he told the patient, or what was in the back of his mind, or what he planned to do at the next visit. Much of this is of short-term value and can be discarded once the episode is over and the summary completed.

A record of drugs prescribed

An accurate record of the dose and quantity of prescribed drugs is of increasing importance – not only for use within the practice, but for medico-legal and research purposes, should an adverse reaction occur.

Nurses and Health Visitors keep records as prescribed by their managers, primarily for monitoring the service being provided. It is the usual practice for team members such as health visitors, district nurses, and midwives to have access to the practice notes, and be encouraged to write in them. Procedures will be needed to ensure that access to records is limited to certain named people, and that confidentiality if preserved.

PROBLEM-ORIENTED MEDICAL RECORDS

Many practices are moving towards problem-oriented records. They provide the doctor with a more logical method, particularly at the stage before a firm diagnosis is made. It helps him to see the patient's problem, as well as to define his own problem, rather than jump to a diagnosis too early.

Problem-oriented records consist of:

(1) identifying particulars and background information (data base);
(2) clinical or progress notes;
(3) the problem list;
(4) the flow chart;
(5) the drug list;

On many records the identifying particulars are faulty, with NHS number or date of birth missing. Full names are essential, with the forename actually used underlined if it is not the first. Particular difficulty may be encountered with Asian names, and this has been well documented by Henley (1979), and simple instructions for receptionists have been published. †

The background information includes significant past illnesses, immunizations, drug or other hypersensitivities, and any special risk factors. It is a permanent and cumulative record which needs to be easily accessible. It is an advantage if it can be copied to be sent with the patient to hospital. In some practices, the patient is shown the data base to ensure its accuracy (often it is

† Obtainable from National Extension College Trust Ltd., 18 Brooklands Avenue, Cambridge, CB2 2HN.
See also Fuller and Toon (1988), see p 275.

not accurate) and to encourage an open attitude between doctor and patient. A questionnaire about health completed by the patient when registering at the practice makes a very good data base. An example is given in Zander *et al.* (1978).

The problem list is a separate sheet of paper on which problems are listed and numbered, with a distinction between active and inactive problems. The progress notes can use the problem number as a sort of shorthand.

The flow chart records a sequence of events, and applies to the supervision of chronic diseases such as hypertension (high blood pressure) or diabetes. Here it is an advantage to have a specially designed form so that key changes are not lost in a morass of progress notes. Antenatal care and child development similarly need flow-charts. The drug list is a flow-chart which is recorded separately.

Further information about A4 or problem-oriented medical records can be obtained from the Information Resources Centre (see Appendix F) or Zander *et al.* (1978). Computerized records are considered in the next chapter. A new series of six booklets on record systems in general practice, by Dr Keith Bolden, is valuable for GPs and practice managers. (Obtainable from Duncan Flockhart Ltd., 700 Oldfield Lane North, Greenford, Middlesex, OB6 0HD.)

ORGANIZING THE MEDICAL RECORD

Each practice must decide whether it wishes to have A4 medical records, the traditional small records, or a mixture of both – for example just transferring the fatter folders to A4.

As well as the blank continuation sheet, various overprinted cards or papers are available for special purpose. For example:

summary sheet;
obstetric record;
child immunization card;
child development record;
contraceptive record;
repeat prescription record;
hypersensitivities;
problem lists;
flow charts;
laboratory report sheets.

Some of this stationery is available from the local FPC, some from the Information Resources Centre, and some is on offer from drug firms. Some practices print or duplicate their own.

The various kinds of printed stationery must be kept in a logical and agreed order, and fastened together by treasury tag, staple, metal clip, glue, or adhesive tape according to preference.

Old continuation sheets can be stapled together and kept at the back of the file, or in a separate pocket. Better still, they can be summarized and then discarded, after removing any identifying details.

Sometimes medical records are packed with blank continuation sheets which have been sent with every change of doctor. These can be thrown away without any qualms.

The most difficult problem with bulky notes is often the thick wad of folded letters and reports. With A4 records they can be filed in date order, with the latest on top. In the older medical records they can be similarly sorted, and secured with a treasury tag. Bulk can be reduced by trimming off surplus paper, or more effectively by discarding duplicate information. When a patient is referred to hospital and admitted, there are often several letters and reports covering the same episode, and duplicating the information. With a policy ruling from the doctor concerned, redundant letters and reports can be destroyed.

Time invested in an efficient record system pays off when the doctor needs to retrieve information about the patient in an emergency. Once the system is designed, staff can work on 'filleting' the records during slack periods. Doctors too can be encouraged not to generate bulky records without good reason, and to throw away redundant information. The records of patients who have died or left the district can be returned to the FPC.

Legibility

For the information contained in the notes to be used it must be legible. The practice manager cannot alter the doctor's handwriting, but she can encourage the doctors to set up a system of typed notes. They can either be written in longhand by the doctor, and typed up immediately after the surgery, or the doctor can dictate notes to be transcribed immediately. Similarly, notes written on visits or night calls can be typed without delay.

Missing notes

Notes can be missing because they have not been received from the FPC. Practices fortunate enough to have a computer can have printed lists of patients' notes not received. Some FPCs will accept a gentle reminder of overdue notes; others will not take kindly to it. However, if notes are needed urgently the doctor may request the FPC to expedite transfer for urgent medical reasons. A telephone call to the previous doctor may be justified in some cases. The problem would be less serious if patients took a note and a summary to their new doctor. It has been strongly argued that patients should be responsible for their own notes. This works well with co-operation cards for obstetric, diabetic, and geriatric patients having shared care. A copy of the summary sheet and data base carried by the patient might be helpful for patients on holiday, and for doctors called in an emergency to a patient they do not know.

Notes can go missing if a doctor has them in the back of his car, or at home, or they are in a pile awaiting letters or research. In extreme cases it may be necessary to mark out borrowed notes like library books, but an eagle-eyed secretary and practice manager will usually know where to find them.

Misfiled notes are also 'missing', and filing is considered next.

STORAGE OF MEDICAL RECORDS

A well-designed filing system is essential to ensure that patients' records can be obtained quickly and accurately. Patient care suffers if notes are not available when needed, or the wrong records have been produced.

The main methods of storage are:

(1) lateral, or shelf filing;
(2) rotary, or carousel filing;
(3) multi drawer cabinets.

More elaborate and expensive systems may be needed where space is limited, such as multi-stack lateral systems on rails, and electrically-operated banks of filing trays. †

Lateral shelving

This uses more space than the other two methods, but has the advantages of easy access and remembering where records are. Misfiling can be reduced by colour-coding the records, and putting a diagonal stripe down the whole section using a felt-tipped pen. Fixed shelving counts as part of the building and is fully reimbursable.

Rotary files

These use space more efficiently than lateral filing, but are more confusing to use, as there are not the same fixed points of reference which guide an experienced clerk around the other systems. It may be helpful to emphasize the starting point of the rotary file with coloured tape or paint, or a clear marker card.

Cabinet files

These may be satisfactory in small practices, but are very time-wasting, and are more likely to cause fatigue or injury to staff than the other systems. They have the advantage that the cabinet can be locked, whereas in the other systems the whole room must be locked.

Guidance about the various filing equipment and methods can be obtained from the Information Resources Centre. In planning a new filing system, plenty of room must be allowed for expansion, both in the bulk of each record and in

† Further information is available in *Medeconomics,* April 1982, pp. 40–47.

the number of records. When expanding premises or moving to a new building, the option of a change to A4 records must be seriously considered, as it may be prevented later by lack of space.

Filing methods

In practices of average size, alphabetical filing is usual, but in large practices sharing a common filing system, there are advantages in a numerical system such as that used in hospitals. Colour coding of records by doctor is all the more important in a large centre.

Family records

There is clear evidence that illness or social problems in one member of a family may cause similar disturbances in other family members, so that a general practitioner may need to diagnose and treat illnesses affecting the family as well as the individuals within it. This task is made easier by a suitable record system.

There are various ways of achieving this. One is to record the family and social history on a family chart (see Zander *et al.* 1978); another is to use an 'F' book or cards (ask Information Resources Centre). Another more elaborate method is to file all the records of one family in a common folder. All these methods require a commitment by the practice to the ideal of family medicine.

CONFIDENTIALITY OF MEDICAL RECORDS AND INFORMATION

Patients, when they come to see a doctor, trust him to keep any confidential information secret. The way in which this trust is maintained depends on every member of the practice staff setting an example, and in the way procedures for handling information are designed and carried out.

The doctors are legally responsible for confidentiality, so a heavy load falls upon them, but they can be helped greatly by policies, rules, and procedures supervised by the practice manager. Mention was made in Chapter 3 of restricting information to those who need to know. Similarly, access to medical records must be subject to strict rules. For example:

Do attached district nurses, health visitors, midwives, and social workers have unrestricted access to patients' notes?
Are they permitted to take them to their own office, or read them in the practice office?
Are medical records of doctors, staff, and their families filed separately under more secure conditions?
Is it possible for cleaners or maintenance staff to gain access to medical records or information?

A balance must be maintained, by mutual trust, between a carefree attitude to confidentiality and an obsession with secrecy which works against the patient's interests. Good procedures will ensure that filing cabinets or rooms are locked at night, and that filing rooms are cleaned only when staff are present. Medical records and reports should not be left unattended in rooms which are not locked at night.

Patients' views on records

Many of the questions raised above can be usefully discussed with a patient group. They tend to trust the doctor implicitly, but are not so keen for their secrets to be open to staff. They mistrust written records to which they themselves do not have access. This objection to their secrets being recorded and passed to other doctors (perhaps with derogatory comments) is understandable. Most doctors write notes on the assumption that patients will not have access to them. If patients had legal right of access to their notes, doctors would perhaps make fewer, or different, notes.

Threats of access to doctors' notes by police and lawyers are very real, and perhaps the time is ripe for the whole question of confidentiality of information to be discussed in practices. The trend towards 'open government' and 'open medicine' are unlikely to be reversed, so it is better to be ready for some changes.

Confidentiality of computer records is now subject to the provisions of the Data Protection Act (1984). All practices holding patient data on computer must register with the Data Protection Registrar (address on p. 273). For a comprehensive file of information apply to the Information Resources Centre (*see* p. 272).

LOGS AND REGISTERS OF PRACTICE ACTIVITY

For any assessment of workload, as well as for efficient day-to-day running of the service, most practices keep a series of log-books to suit their particular needs and circumstances. Some examples are listed below:

(1) log of patients seen by each doctor;
(2) log of home visits by each doctor;
(3) register of hospital appointments requested;
(4) register of hospital transport requests;
(5) register of X-rays requested;
(6) list (on notice board or white board) of patients in hospital;
(7) register of deaths;
(8) day-book for recording messages (see Chapter 3);
(9) log of practice nurse's workload.

The log of patients seen by each doctor each day can be taken from the appointment book sheets. Before they are removed from the book the total can be totted up and entered in the log. At the end of each month the numbers of sessions, and patients seen can be summarized, and shown to the partners. This device provides hard facts about workload, to dispel any myths about who is working hardest! But numbers of patients seen is a poor measure of effectiveness of health care. First-attendances and repeat visits can be logged separately, to provide further clues.

New home visits can be logged from the day book or visiting list; repeat visits can be abstracted by the secretary from the doctor's diary.

A register of hospital appointments requested is a valuable check on the efficiency of the hospital clerical system. If a patient does not receive an appointment by post, the book provides evidence that one was requested. If there are columns for urgency of request (e.g. within 14 days) and the date the patient is seen is filled in later, then valuable evidence of the responsiveness of the various hospital departments can be collected, which can be used to bring pressure on the laggards. Referral rates can also be calculated, but to be complete they must include details of emergency referrals, not just the 'cold' referrals.

A register of hospital transport requests will be useful if angry patients complain that transport did not come.

A register of X-ray requests can be incorporated in the hospital appointment register in a small practice.

The list of patients in hospital has already been mentioned as an aid to the doctor and other staff to visit them or keep in touch. A more permanent record of numbers in hospital, though subject to many confounding factors, does give a measure of the effectiveness of the practice and the community in caring for people at home.

A small book to register all the patients of the practice who die can be kept in the reception office, so that all doctors and staff can see it. This can prove a valuable way to communicate with other team members, so that they do not visit relatives thinking that the patient is still alive. It is a starting point for bereavement counselling by various team members, and a reminder for anniversary visits.

The day book for recording messages has been mentioned on p. 48 as a useful way for team members to communicate, and as a permanent medicolegal record.

The practice nurse is wise to log her workload, under various headings, so that annual statistics can be prepared to monitor the trends. This topic is dealt with in more detail in Pritchard (1981), *Manual of primary health care*.

This list is not complete, but can be a starting point for the practice manager or secretary in designing her own logging and monitoring system. It is not enough just to put data into books. To be useful, it needs to be summarized, distributed, and discussed. The practice newsletter described in Chapter 3 is one way of disseminating the information. Another is for the practice manager, with the support of the partners and other staff, to produce an annual report of the activities of the practice. This is hard work, but so is all monitoring!

AN INFORMATION SYSTEM FOR GENERAL PRACTICE

The medical record is an important part of the overall information system for general practice. What does the system have to do? The basic raw material in an average practice of 2331 patients is:

consultations per annum	8857
other items of service (e.g. prescriptions, telephone contacts)	15 082
laboratory tests	406
X-ray reports	1239
referrals to hospital	336
admissions to hospital	257

at a total cost to the Exchequer of £216 852 (Metcalfe 1982).

As well as coping with this considerable demand, the record has to serve the needs of:

(1) preventive medicine – at risk groups;
(2) quality control – patient recall, performance review;
(3) practice planning, administration, and finance;
(4) education – doctor, staff, trainee, patients;
(5) research.

This can be shown graphically (Fig. 11.1) as an interaction between doctor (backed by team and NHS resources) and patient (as part of a registered population). The medical record logs this interaction.

The age–sex register

The practice population can be better served by an age–sex register to help identify people at risk.

Much is talked about this new status-symbol for high quality general practice, but what does it aim to achieve, and are these aims realized? First what is it? The medical record cards are usually filed alphabetically, so to select all the people called Jones or Brown, is easy. If we wish to make a list of all those over 85, or females coming up to their 35th birthday in the next three months, then we have a difficult job. If we make a card out for everyone on the list (of different colour for males and females) including name, address, and date of birth, and arrange these in birth-date order, then it is a matter of minutes to select those in the age group required.

Once an age–sex register is constructed, it must be kept up to date by removing cards from the index of patients who have left the list or died, and making out new cards for new arrivals, including births. In some inner-city practices with a turnover approaching 25 per cent per annum this is a formidable task. Ways of extending the range of the register to include things like social class, ethnic background, or occupation are considered under computers. Index cards can be obtained from the Information Resources Centre.

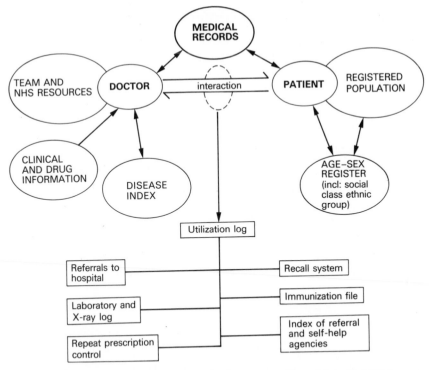

Fig. 11.1. Model of a medical information system. (From Metcalfe 1982.)

Once we have an age–sex register, what use is it?

(1) checking child health screening or immunization of children up to age 5;

(2) checking rubella immunization of 11-year-old girls;

(3) preparing lists for cervical screening of women aged 35–65 (five-year intervals);

(4) preparing lists for hypertension screening;

(5) preparing lists of the elderly for geriatric surveys, or surveillance by health visitors;

(6) preparing an age–sex profile of the practice (see p. 169).

Unless there is active preventive medicine or research taking place in the practice, the labour of preparing the register is not cost-effective.

The disease index (diagnostic index)

This is a list of all the patients who have certain diseases which are of interest to the practice; or it can include all recorded diagnoses or problems. The latter is more extensive and complete, but contains much information which is not actually used. It is a good general rule not to collect useless information, which clutters up the system, and makes retrieval of essential data more difficult. At its simplest, notes can be colour-tagged according to the RCGP (1964) system:

Red   Allergy or hypersensitivity
Blue   Hypertension
Green   Tuberculosis
Yellow   Epilepsy
Black   Suicide risk
White   Long-term therapy (e.g. steroids, hormones, etc.)
Orange   Diabetes
(Other colours or patterns may be added at will for use in the practice.)

For greater detail an 'E' book is needed. This is a loose-leaf ledger with a separate leaf for each disease. As a patient attends, his name is filled in by the doctor on the appropriate diagnostic page. Alternatively a trained clerk can do it from the notes. Details of this method can be obtained from the Information Resources Centre (see p. 272). Like age-sex registers, the disease index is more suitable for a computer system, which is considered later.

CLINICAL AND DRUG INFORMATION

A general practitioner cannot keep all the information he needs in his head, nor can he update his memory satisfactorily, because of the explosive growth of knowledge. He must back up his memory with a good information system. Drug information has already been considered (see p. 135). Information about diseases and their treatment may come from many sources, for example:

memories or notes from medical school or post-graduate lectures;
consultants' recommendations;
medical journals;
textbooks;
drug company promotion;
government publications and NHS circulars;
audio or video cassettes;
computerized data systems.

Each doctor has his individual system, but the practice manager may have a part to play in making information accessible when it is needed. This applies in particular to journals, text books, and government publications. Computer systems will be considered later. First let us consider the use of libraries.

LIBRARIES

Clinical information can be available in the practice in the form of text books, journals, reprints, and circulars, or it can be obtained from outside libraries, at for example:

postgraduate centre;
district hospital;
regional health authority;
DHSS;
Kings Fund Centre;
Royal College of General Practitioners;
British Medical Association;
Royal Society of Medicine and other Medical Societies;
Local Authority public libraries, backed by British Library Service.

The last four are available only to members. Most will lend books, and will supply photocopies of journal articles on request. Some will do a computerized literature search such as *Medline*. Most computer and library systems are based on USA classifications in which general practice appears only as a professional activity, not as a branch of medicine having its own body of knowledge. So libraries geared to the needs of general practice (such as RCGP and BMA) may be more appropriate.

The RCGP library produces a regular bibliography, listing all available text books and journal articles by subject and author, and also topic bibliographies which include practice administration as well as clinical matters. The DHSS Library holds an on-line computerized database called DHSS-Data which can be accessed through medical libraries. Direct access is possible but expensive.

The practice library

General practitioners have not been prominent in the past as either authors or as buyers of textbooks, but this is changing rapidly under the influence of vocational training. What should the practice library cover, and what would this cost? Libraries should not be measured in numbers of titles or in cost, but in the way they serve the information needs of the practice. So what are the information needs?

Reference works needed urgently: 'bench books'

Drug information has been considered already. Information about emergencies, text books of medicine, surgery, obstetrics, gynaecology, paediatrics, dermatology, etc, and on treatment (therapeutics) need to be at hand. Many doctors like to have these at home as personal reference works in emergency, or at weekends. Some may also be needed at the practice, or even in individual doctor's consulting rooms.

Reference works and monographs needed less urgently

There is no point in having books on the shelf which are not used, and conversely, if key information is not available when needed the patient will suffer. A number of books may be of value, and the RCGP has a good bibliography – particularly for teaching practices (see Appendix F for address).

The method of acquiring books for the library is important. If all partners have to agree before a book is bought the library will be small, as their information needs differ. The practice manager may be the best person to hold the library budget, and to order the books on request from partners or trainee up to that total. If the budget is likely to be exceeded, she can try to raise extra funds (e.g. from drug firms). She can also keep a balance between the various partners' appetite for books.

The doctors have a responsibility for providing books needed in the treatment room. But district nurses and health visitors like to have access to medical books; they also need some books of their own. It is unlikely that NHS funds will be forthcoming, so it is an opportunity for the partners to make a generous gesture towards team working, by including books needed by nurses and other staff in the budget. A display of new books and current journals in the staff room is a good start.

But more important than books and journals is a system which will ensure that appropriate information is available when and where it is needed. This is considered next in connection with journals and circulars which arrive in such enormous quantity, that there is no question of reading them all, let alone remembering the important details.

Journal articles and circulars

Should old journals be kept, or just the articles thought to be useful? If the journals are kept, they will have to be stored neatly and in order, and the indices kept together for quick reference. Useful articles can be emphasized on the contents page for quick recall.

Alternatively, useful papers can be torn out and filed under subject. A system is needed to ensure that one is not just collecting useless paper.

If the practice is prepared to invest in information from this source, a key-word system can be adopted. The doctor reading the journal marks the articles he wants indexed, and underlines words in the title which he regards as key words. For example, in an article on 'Anti-smoking education in general practice' he would probably underline *smoking*, and add *health* to *education* and underline them. The secretary makes out a card with the author(s) name, title, and reference – just as the references in this book. The key words can be underlined or added. Each new card is given a number in serial order. These cards are kept alphabetically by author in a small index file. There is a separate file of key words, also in alphabetical order. If the keyword chosen does not appear, a new card is made out. The serial number is put on the key-word card, and also on the torn-out or photocopied article. The articles are filed by serial number in box files. To find a reference to a topic – look in the keyword file, and retrieve the article from the box file. An article by a particular author can be found by first obtaining the number from the alphabetical reference file, and then going to the box file.

There are more complex ways of filing where the number of references is large. For a full description of this system, the 'accession number indexing system', see de Alarcon (1969). Larger systems can best be computerized.

Advice from librarian

We have already mentioned that books for instant use should be available where they are needed – for example, at the doctor's home, the trainee's consulting room, the treatment room, and the prescribing desk. These are the 'bench-books'. A main practice library will need to be accessible to all, so its siting will depend on the layout of the surgery or health centre. If there is a staff common room, this might be ideal.

Before setting up any library or information system, it is essential to get advice from a professional librarian. Such advice can be obtained from the postgraduate centre or district hospital librarian. More specific general practice information can be obtained from the librarian at the RCGP (address on p. 272). It is unlikely that an international classification will be needed for a practice library, and a professional librarian will be able to suggest a simpler system. Few practices can afford a librarian – their salaries cannot be re-imbursed.

If a practice secretary looks after the library, she can be briefed by the local librarian. If the librarian can be coaxed into visiting the practice, his or her advice would be invaluable. Particular issues on which advice are needed are the proportion of money to spend on books as against labour in retrieving information; and ways of selecting the most relevant information source from the mass of data showered upon the GP – much of it from drug companies. A friendly librarian can save the general practitioner from 'information overkill'.

Practice manager's information needs

Drug firms help to fill the large gap in administrative and financial information, by their excellent publications on 'the business of general practice', *Pulse blue book, General Practitioner 'In practice'* supplements, and *'Medeconomics'*. All of these make the practice manager's task much easier. She too needs her 'bench books' which would feature these, as well as the 'Red Book'. Other publications she might need for reference are listed below:

Gann, R. (1981). *Help for health*. Information for primary care. Wessex regional library unit. Southampton General Hospital, Southampton SO9 4XY.
Help for health is a pioneer scheme to help primary care professionals obtain all the information they need about services available for patients. Though designed to serve the Wessex region, it has a comprehensive list of national organizations. Other regions are hoping to follow the Wessex model.
Jones, R. V. H. *et al.* (1985). *Running a practice*. 3rd Edn. Croom Helm, London.
Locke, M. (1980). *How to run committees and meetings*. Papermac.
Parr, C. W. and Williams, J. P. (1981). *Family practitioner services and their administration*. Institute of Health Service Administration, 75 Portland Place, London W1N 4AN.

Pritchard, P. (1981). *Manual of primary health care,* 2nd Edn. Oxford University Press, Oxford.
Winthrop. *The general practitioner's yearbook.* (Ed. D. A. E. Lansdell.) Parts 1 and 2 (1983). Winthrop Laboratories, Surbiton, Surrey.

A list of books on management for further reading is included as Appendix G.

INFORMATION FOR PATIENTS

Handouts for patients about the services available have been described in Chapter 8. Information about health has been considered in Chapters 7 and 11. Letting the patient see his own 'data base' and check its accuracy was mentioned earlier in this chapter. An even more drastic step has been to give patients access to medical information in the form of a patients' library. This has been tried and found to be popular. It has worked in predominantly working class areas, and it has not been abused, or caused any friction.

In addition to straight medical text books, there are now a number of texts written mostly by doctors specifically for patients and these would be very suitable for such a library. If the budget does not cover these, then voluntary subscriptions might be invited. An alternative is to have a handout with the list of titles, so that the patient may order them from the public library. A selection of titles is given in Appendix E.

12 Computers

The very word conjures up an image of a future world with all drudgery banished, or alternatively a present world where things are unnecessarily complex, and the computer gets the blame. How can we reap the benefits without the frustrations?

Buying a computer is not like buying a washing machine – just install it, read the instructions, and press the button. It is more like engaging a new and highly proficient member of staff, to do new as well as old tasks, but who speaks in a language that has to be learnt.

WHAT IS A COMPUTER?

Much hard work and thinking is needed before buying a computer, or failure is assured. So first let us ask ourselves what a computer is and what it does. Literally, it is a machine which does sums, but today we mean a machine which stores and analyses information, and then retrieves it in a more useful form – that is to say 'data processing'. the quality of the output depends on the quality of the input (the human factor), the efficiency and scope of the machine (hardware), and the effectiveness of the instructions given to the machine (software). Hence the jocular 'GIGO effect' – garbage in: garbage out.

There are many unfamiliar terms whose meaning must be learnt. Some will be described here, but for a fuller glossary of computer terms the reader should turn to some of the books quoted at the end of the chapter.

The actual machinery of the computer is called *hardware*. This consists of an *input* (usually modified typewriter keyboard), a *processing unit*, a *memory unit*, and *output* in the form of *visual display units* (VDUs; like a television screen) and a *printer* or printers (see note on p. 166). The processing unit can be a *microcomputer*, which is usually desk-top size and relatively cheap. Several can be linked together in one practice, if the capacity of one unit is not enough.

Memory is needed of the data which is being processed (e.g. the names, addresses, and dates of birth of all the practice patients). On small 'hobby' microcomputers the memory can be an ordinary cassette tape, but this is unlikely to be enough for the needs of a practice. There is a choice of *floppy disks* which have a moderate memory capacity,† and *hard disks* which have a

---

†Memory in a computer is measured in *bytes*. A byte is a letter or number built up from several *bits*, which are the basic electrical unit in a computer, representing a binary digit (0 or 1). A 5¼ in. floppy disk can hold upwards of 100 000 bytes (100 KB or kilo-bytes). A dual density floppy disk can hold a million bytes (1 MB or megabyte). Hard disks have the advantages of greater memory and faster access times, but they are more expensive.

much greater memory and are better for the larger practice making full use of a computer. They are a bit like gramophone records, and are operated in a *disk drive unit*. The disks are changed by hand. Usually one disk or set of disks, is used for memory; and a second for the instructions for the computer – the program, or *software*. Hence the need for a double disk-drive unit.

Larger than the microcomputer is the *minicomputer*, with greater capacity; but it is more expensive. Several practices might share a remote computer, with a *terminal* (such as a VDU) in the practice and connected by telephone line. This central computer might be a minicomputer, or an even larger '*mainframe*' computer, such as that operated by a health authority or commercial computer bureau. These have vast memory stores – some on hard disk, some on tape – and formidable data processing power. Different users would share the time available for computer use, and be charged accordingly. Not everyone could use the computer at once, so it might not be possible to obtain an instant response (as required to show what drugs a patient is taking) at peak times. The alternative to instant response from the computer (*real time*) is to have *batches* of data processed by the mainframe computer when it is not so busy, for example at night. This is a very economical way of processing data. Input can be by proformas completed by the practice staff. Output can be in the form of practice lists, schedules of appointments for recall, etc. An example of this kind of usage is the immunization programme for children run by many health authorities. However, it has problems of remoteness, risk to confidentiality, and slow response. While it is not satisfactory for things like prescription writing, it is probably still the cheapest option for lists of practice patients.

However, the trend is very much away from the large mainframe computer and towards the 'in house' microcomputer, so this will be the main emphasis of this chapter.

Confidentiality is better assured by an 'in house' system, but in general, confidential data is safer in a computer than in manual systems, and security checks can be built in to computer programs to make sure of this (*see* p. 156).

Printers

Computers generate a lot of paper with typed characters on it. If there is any point in the exercise at all, then someone has to read the printed output, or at least refer to it. For legibility, the type quality needs to be good. There are many makes and types of printer, and in general you get what you pay for. The cheaper printers use a 'dot-matrix', where each character is made up of a series of dots. They are not so easy to read and are less suitable for 'letter quality' output. For these a proper typeface is needed – usually a 'daisy-wheel' printer or the familiar golf ball. There are many other varieties, of which details may be sought in *Which computer* magazine. It is likely that the supplier of a general practice computer system (hardware + software) will have a range of printers to choose from. If two printers are needed, one – say for prescriptions – could be a dot matrix printer, and the second a daisy wheel machine for listings and possibly for letters (see Chapter 15). All printers are noisy, and if they cannot have a room or sound-proof cubicle to themselves, then they can be silenced by a sound-proof box. Printers vary in their speed, and in the number of characters per line (from about 80 to over 200).

Computers are no panacea, but they are very powerful and efficient clerks and helpers if used properly. In this chapter we will consider ways in which computers can help in general practice and the implications for management of using one.

WHAT CAN A COMPUTER DO WELL?

First we must ask ourselves 'what tasks do we have in running the practice, or providing patient care, which a computer *could do better than a manual system?*' Like must be compared with like, namely an efficient manual system compared with an efficient computer. Sometimes manual systems are cheaper and easier to run, at less cost and effort. Examples are the daily appointment book, oral contraceptive recalls, and child immunization (Appendix A). These could all be computerized, but would it be worth the effort and cost? If someone else is paying, then that is a different matter!

Having made a list of practice problems which data-processing might solve, we must put the possible uses in a logical order, because some uses are basic to any system and should be done first. We then have a list from which to choose those uses which we want and can afford now, and those which can wait. Not all the partners may have the same ideas, so flexibility and compromise are needed from the start to include the different requirements, some of which may conflict.

An example of such a list follows, and is based on Metcalfe (1982) and Lucas and Metcalfe (1982) which should be consulted at the outset:

(1) basic practice register, with listings as needed, such as age–sex register;
(2) diagnostic or problem index, and patient surveillance;
(3) prescription writing and monitoring;
(4) 'Look-up' data systems such as drug information, clinical and library information, Prestel, etc.;
(5) 'Question and answer' systems for patients, doctors, and staff;
(6) fully computerized medical records.

More details of these uses are given in Table 12.1, and in succeeding paragraphs. They are examples, and are not intended to be comprehensive. Computerizing the practice accounts, and using a computer as a word processor, are dealt with in Chapters 13 and 15.

The time-scale for deciding on a computer and installing it is much longer than most people, and salesmen, imagine. The lesson is to spend a year or two in deciding, and then probably implement the plan in stages. In parallel, the existing manual systems can be sorted out and made more efficient, so that the

Table 12.1. *Check list of possible computer uses*

Main category of use	Essential data	Optional extra data	Output	Batch/† real time
1. Basic practice register	name; address; sex; date of birth	Person number, NHS number, date registered, doctor with whom registered, doctor usually seen, telephone number, postcode, title/marital status, number in household, social class, occupation, ethnic group	Practice list; list by doctor; lists for child health surveillance, rubella immunization, cervical, and hypertension screening; lists of 65–74 and over 75-year-olds; check of list numbers; population histogram; printed labels	Batch
2. Diagnostic or problem index and patient surveillance	Diagnosis or problem (coded) against name or person number and date	Date last seen, date of next appointment; medical summaries, data base; consultation data	Diagnostic lists; recall system; clinic schedules; lists of defaulters; printed labels; risk factors; item of service claims; copies of data base; work load statistics	Batch
3. Prescription writing and monitoring	Name and address (or person number); age; drug name (coded), dose, quantity; number of repeats allowed	Drug hypersensitivities and contraindications; drug incompatibilities and interactions; link up with drug information system; oral contraceptive data	Initial prescriptions; repeat prescriptions; warnings of interactions, side effects, hypersensitivity; item of service claims etc., statistics of prescribing by drug/category/cost	Real time
4. 'Look up' data systems	Information from bureau by telephone line, or by locally held disk, or via television channels		Drug information system; clinical information; library service; Prestel, etc.	Real time
5. Question and answer systems	Computer link with information service, or locally-held disk or program		Computer-assisted diagnosis; prompts; patient questionnaires; health education; risk analysis	Real time
6. Fully computerized medical records	Basic file; data base; problem summary; narrative record and prescription file		Direct interaction by doctor (and patient) with information system	Real time

† Batch mode. Forms are completed in the practice and sent weekly to a (mainframe) computer, which then processes it and returns the results later to the user. Real-time. The user is in contact with the computer which processes that data as it is fed in.

transfer of data to the computer is as smooth as possible. It is easier for beginners to improve a manual system, rather than to do it while involved in computerization. The worst option is to computerize faulty data, and then try to sort it out!

Basic practice register

All general practice data systems start with the list of practice patients – similar to the list held on index-cards by the Family Practitioner Committee.† The essential data are the surname, forenames, date of birth, and sex of patients. It is helpful to have in addition their title (Mr/Mrs/Miss/Ms), the date of registration, NHS number, doctor with whom registered, and doctor usually seen (UD). Some systems use a personal number for ease of access to the computer. All this information can just be squeezed on to one line of wide (39 cm) computer print-out. If the half-width paper is used, then another method is needed, such as identifying people by surname and date of birth, and calling up full information if required.

Some practices find other data useful, such as telephone number, post code, and so on (see Table 12.1). The temptation to put all the available data on to the computer must be resisted by remembering the labour and cost of collecting, storing, and updating such data, and asking oneself how often it will actually be used.

The uses of the basic data file are legion. Reception staff and secretaries find it handy to have an up-to-date alphabetical list of patients at their elbow. It makes it possible to have a much tidier record system. Each doctor can have a list of his personal patients (both registered and those usually seen). Lists of, for example, those aged over 65 are also helpful for the health visitors. Lists of females of an age to need rubella vaccination or cervical screening, and lists produced for child-health or hypertension screening can be valuable. They can be in monthly batches if this is more convenient for scheduling screening clinics.

It is normally unnecessary to print out the age–sex register (i.e. the practice list in birth order) as a whole, but it can be summarized on one sheet of paper, automatically printed by the computer, as a population histogram or practice profile. This is useful for assessing the distribution of population in the practice (and by doctor) and for observing changes in the pattern which may have planning implications.

The basic practice register, once completed, must be kept up-to-date by adding new arrivals, deleting those who have left the list; and changing names, addresses, and marital status and so on. In practices with a high turnover, this is a major task. Easy-to-operate systems must be devised so that the changes are

---

†Some FPCs are at last transferring to computers so might be able to help the practice develop the basic register. If the two systems are compatible, the FPC could supply the practice register on disk or by direct line which could be fed into the practice computer at regular intervals.

recorded. Only one entry should be needed to change the basic register and its subfiles and to inform the FPC. If money allows, the printing of sticky labels can make transfer to A4 files and changing address much easier. Labels can be time-saving for laboratory and X-ray forms, FPC claims forms, and for sending for patients for screening. Lists can be made of patients whose medical records have not arrived at intervals of one, two or three months after registration. Total list numbers can be provided quarterly, as well as those of patients aged over 65 and 75, as a rough check on FPC capitation payments.

Diagnostic or problem-index and patient surveillance

The next stage, for which many practices will opt, is to identify those patients with special problems or risk factors, or who need careful surveillance. Examples are patients:

who smoke cigarettes;
with:
  hypertension;
  diabetes;
  epilepsy;
  alcohol problems;
  drug abuse;
  hypersensitivities;
  rheumatoid arthritis;
  other chronic diseases;
  other risk factors;
on:
  steroids;
  hormone-replacement therapy;
  oral contraceptives.

Each practice, or each doctor, may have his own list of interesting diagnoses. As well as listing those who need surveillance, it is a small step to develop a recall system so that patients who do not attend when they should are listed and sent reminders. This ensures that surveillance is 'fail-safe', as far as is humanly possible. It is usual to use a standard code for diagnoses or problems, e.g. OXMIS or RCGP code.† The OXMIS problem code book lists alphabetically all possible diagnoses or problems likely to be encountered in general practice, and gives them a code of up to six digits or letters. For example, abdominal pain is coded as 7855D, zoster (herpes) is 053. It also gives the RCGP code (usually four digit) and the International (ICHPPC) code (up to eight digits). The OXMIS code has the advantage of being more comprehensive than the RCGP code, and less complicated than the ICHPPC code, for use

†OXMIS problem codes 1978 obtainable from OXMIS, P.O. Box 77, Headington, Oxford, OX3 7UG.
RCGP code, obtainable from Royal College of General Practitioners, 14 Princes Gate, London, SW7 1PU, but is also included in the OXMIS code book.

of which staff usually need special training. The point of coding is that computer space is saved and classification is more logical, so that information can be retrieved more accurately.

The next step is a larger one, to ensure that all important medical history and data are recorded on the computer, so that problem lists and summary print-outs may be kept up-to-date and put in the record as part of the data-base. Whereas the basic practice register ask little of the doctor, the diagnostic index and surveillance scheme require him to behave in a systematic way, which may not be easy when he is under pressure. Completing summaries and data-bases for all patients is a major labour of love – though parts of it can be delegated, at a cost.

There are two ways of feeding information into such a system. One is for the doctor to enter all the diagnoses/problems in which he is interested on to a pro-forma, which is fed into the computer. The other is to enter all doctor/patient encounters and diagnoses/problems. This can be done by a trained clerk. Recording all encounters is a more 'fail-safe' system, but is more expensive and can fill up the computer memory with unwanted data. As computers become cheaper, encounter records could become feasible, and would automatically generate work-load and activity statistics.

In all the systems considered so far, data can be processed by a computer in batches, so it is possible to use a remote computer or bureau, and money is saved by not requiring the computer to work in 'real-time'. With the development of modern microcomputers with substantial memory, housed in the practice, the distinction becomes less important.

Prescription-writing and monitoring

Much doctor and staff time is spend writing prescriptions, which cost as much as the general practitioner service. Doctors get little feedback about their pre-scribing and the consequences of errors are serious.

Very successful systems have been devised for prescription-writing, and this can automatically generate the statistics needed to monitor prescribing. The DHSS has produced FP10s in a format which can be used in the printer of a computer.

There are three essentials for such a system to operate conveniently:

1. It must be a real-time system.

2. The terminal, and preferably the printer, should be on the doctor's desk.

3. A separate printer is needed to save changing the paper whenever a pre-scription is issued.

Though prescriptions can be typed in plain English, much time can be saved by using a drug code. Each doctor can construct his own 'minicopoeia' and code, but a standard code such as the OCHP† is preferable, so that staff can use it

† Details may be obtained from the Oxford Community Health Project, Old Road, Headington, Oxford, OX3 7LF.

for repeat prescriptions. The Prescription Pricing Authority has a complete code of all prescribable drugs, which can be made available.

A drug interaction program can be added so that the doctor will be warned of potential interactions or contraindications – for example, which drugs should not be given in pregnancy.

Regular statistics of prescribing of individual drugs and groups of drugs can be provided for each doctor or practice and compared against the national figures of drugs used and of cost. Dispensing practices can use the computer for stock control.

'Look-up' and data systems

Already drug-information systems are available which will give detailed information about drugs on request. These include *Prestel* and other experimental systems to which access can be obtained by telephone line. Similar systems are being developed for clinical information and library references, so that one day text books may become obsolete. If the data bank is large, the computer would be remotely sited; smaller amounts of data could be held on disk and used in the practice (e.g. drug interaction).

Question and answer systems

In these the doctor (or manager or patient) interacts with the computer. Such programs can be used to help a doctor arrive at a diagnosis, or the patient to give a history. They have been used successfully, but are in an early stage of development. A promising development is the use of educational programs by patients to help them assess their own health risks and promote their own health.

Fully computerized medical records

This system can allow the doctor (with a computer terminal on his desk) to dispense with paper, medical records, or even his pen. It has been used successfully in Exeter, but requires great enthusiasm from the GPs, and is expensive. A computer breakdown is more serious in this type of system. It may well be the method of the future, but it is probably best for practices to start with the uses listed 1–3 (Table 12.1) and graduate to full computerization only when they have had thorough experience of the simpler systems. By then the art will have developed even further, so that predicting future outcomes is difficult. The combination of a rapidly developing computer market, and the changes in behaviour brought about by using computers, makes it essential that the system chosen should be versatile and expandable. We have to learn to live with objectives that are over the horizon, such is the speed of change.

IMPLICATIONS FOR MANAGEMENT OF COMPUTERIZATION

So far there has been little mention of buying a computer. That comes later. Having surveyed what computers can do, the doctors and staff must discuss which tasks to computerize. Before deciding on the options, it is advisable for the manager to work out what data might be needed, and whether it is available. A computer will concentrate the mind, but will not turn messy data into good data. An important question is how good are the practice data, and can they be improved? For example, how many records are missing, relate to people who have left, have not date of birth or NHS number, have incorrect addresses or names? How many notes contain information about immunization, sensitivities, summary of major illnesses, records of blood pressure, cigarette smoking or current medication?

A start can be made by checking for missing data every time a patient appears at the desk, and finally marking the notes if it is all complete. Progress can be checked with a target date for completion well in advance of the arrival of the computer.

Doctors and staff will need to change their behaviour, both to introduce a computer and to keep using it. Has this behaviour been specified in detail, and will the doctors and staff live up to their promises? Enough flexibility will be needed to cover different levels of commitment and disagreements. Have doctors and staff visited a practice with a comparable system working? Have any of them tried a 'hobby' computer at home?

Detailed work will be needed before deciding on which programs to introduce. Priorities must be agreed; and costing both in money and staff-time set out in detail. Should the programme be implemented all at once, or can it be phased? What staff training will be needed? Is this included in the package? When a short list of options and priorities has been drawn up, the suppliers can go into more detail about software (programs) and hardware (equipment) needed to carry them out. The emphasis now is on micro-computers, in the practice, and with hard disk memory. Only a small number of firms has developed programs for general practice, but they use commercial equipment, details of which may be checked in periodicals like *Which Computer*.

Many other questions need to be asked, such as reliability of equipment (and of the firm supplying it), its useful life, maintenance costs, quick availability of maintenance, procedures when equipment is not working, and so on. Reference should be made to the books listed, or to an experienced user to refine the check list. Not until then will a decision be considered on which equipment and software to buy. It is a long and difficult road, but with a very satisfactory outcome if successful. A check list follows:

Check list for practice managers considering computerization in their practice

1. What are the problems in running the practice, and providing medical care?

2. Would a computerized data processing system be more effective than a manual system?

3. Is the present system as efficient as possible?

4. What can be done now to improve the quality of the data, so that any future transition to computerization is smoother?

5. Which of the possible computer uses would the practice like to develop, and in what order of priority?

6. Has all possible advice been sought – from experienced users, RCGP, RHA, FPC, etc?

7. What will be the requirements in capital cost, maintenance, staff time, staff training, doctor time, and change in doctor's behaviour?

8. Is there an adequate level of agreement between partners?

9. What software and hardware options are available and which is the chosen system? Is it easy to use, flexible, and expandable.

10. Does the firm provide staff training, after-sales maintenance, and advice? At what cost?

11. Is the firm financially secure?

12. Can the equipment link up with outside data systems?

13. What is the total cost of the system chosen (capital and revenue).

14. What is the time scale of implementation and obsolescence?

15. Is confidentiality of patient records assured?

Further reading

Malcolm, A. and Poyser, J. (eds) (1982). Computers and the general practitioner. Pergamon Press, Oxford, for Royal College of General Practitioners.

RCGP (1980). *Computers in primary care.* Report of Computer Working Party. Occasional Paper No. 13. Royal College of General Practitioners.

Sheldon, M. and Stoddart, N. (1985). *Trends in general practice computing.* Royal College of General Practitioners, London.

Coding books

ICHPPC-2-Defined. (1983). *International classification of health problems in primary care.* 3rd Edn. Oxford University Press, Oxford.

IC-Process-PC (1986). *International classifications of process in primary care.* Oxford University Press, Oxford.

ICPC (1988) *International classification of primary care.* Oxford University Press.

Computer Society

Primary Health Care Specialist Group of the British Computer Society. Secretary: Dr Nick Robinson, 4 Aldery Avenue, Hounslow, Middlesex, TW5 0QL. Tel: 01 577 5431.

13 Finance

Financial decisions must be taken by the partners, who are in effect the directors and shareholders of the business. The practice manager's role is crucial in ensuring that the partners have the best information on which to make decisions, and that the financial affairs of the practice run smoothly. The practice must make a profit, out of which the partners are remunerated, and future developments financed. The profit is the difference between income and expenditure, so to maximize profit, income must be as great as possible, and expenditure controlled.

Remuneration of GPs is very complex, but it is all worked out with the aim of an average gross NHS remuneration per partner of £42 219, and average expenses of £13 480 resulting in an average net remuneration of £28 800.† Thus expenses are about 33 per cent of the gross income. This is an average figure and expenses fall equally on each side of the average. Practices which have expenses of less than £13 480 (or 33 per cent) may be providing a relatively poor service; practices with expenses above that level may offer patients a lavish service at the expense of the partners 'take-home pay'. This dilemma is built in to the system. Doctors mostly prefer to work in good conditions with ample staff, but they may be poorer for it.

The practice manager must ensure that revenue (both NHS and non-NHS) is maximized, and that expenditure is cost-effective and not wasteful. If she can keep the practice profit well above the average, then more money will be available for services for patients and staff, without impoverishing the partners.

The Review Body which advises on general practitioners' pay takes into account the expenses actually incurred by practices (from a sample of income-tax returns), so if all doctors doubled their payments to staff, they would be none the poorer for it – after a delay of two years. Equally, if all doctors doubled the number of 'item of service claims' they would be none the richer in the long run, as these payments are taken into account in calculating the average net remuneration. It is an uphill struggle to keep ahead of the field, which can tax the skill of partners, practice manager, and accountant. Some hints will be given in this chapter under the headings:

1. Revenue – generating revenue, NHS and non-NHS.
2. Expenditure – cost-effectiveness.
3. Income tax – minimizing tax liability.

†1988 figures; for up-to-date figures see *Medeconomics*.

4. Capital – finance of buildings, equipment, cars, etc.

5. Financial management – keeping accounts, information for management and planning, financial control.

6. Computerization of practice accounts.

REVENUE

Revenue from the NHS

The bulk of practice revenue comes from the NHS – in most practices, less than 10 per cent is non-NHS revenue. The practice receives a quarterly statement from the FPC which lists the various heads of revenue, and deductions, and sends a cheque to the practice, usually on 1 January, April, July, and October. A monthly advance can be paid on request, which greatly eases the cash flow. Most of the payments are quarterly in arrears, but the counting date (e.g. of claim forms) is usually stated, so that the figures may be checked. The quarterly statement is a most valuable document which forms the basis for the analysis of revenue from the NHS. The form may vary between different FPCs and Health Boards, but the information given is similar. As well as the income from various sources, it lists deductions such as superannuation, loan repayments, or health-centre charges.

The fees and allowances come within various categories which are given in detail in the 'Red Book' (*Statement of fees and allowances*). They are reprinted in a handy form in *Medeconomics*, and *The GP Pocket Guide to The Red Book* 1988/9. The categories are summarized below:

(1) basic practice allowances;
(2) capitation fees;
(3) item of service fees;
(4) other allowances and payments from FPC;
(5) NHS income separate from FPCs.

These fees and allowances will be considered in turn in the context of the practice manager's role. Reimbursement of certain practice expenses will be considered later.

Basic practice allowances

These allowances represent a fixed part of the doctor's pay, which is needed as a minimum for running a practice of over 1000 patients. It cannot, by statute, exceed half the GP's pay. There are additional allowances for leave, group practice, seniority, vocational training, out-of-hours service, for practising in a designated area, and for employing an assistant. The qualifying conditions for these allowances are set out in the 'Red Book', and normally their payment presents no problem. The finance officer of the FPC will explain any apparent anomalies.

One cautionary note relates to designated area allowances. These are payments to attract a doctor to underdoctored areas, and provide an incentive to introduce another partner. However, the introduction of another partner may result in the area no longer being designated, so that several practices may lose their allowances after three years. Close liaison with the FPC, Local Medical Committee, and other practices should get round the difficulty.

Capitation fees

These fees are paid in respect of each patient on the list, and so give extra fees to those with a larger case load. There is a basic capitation fee (currently £8.25) for those under the age of 65. A larger fee is paid for patients between 65 and 74, and 75 years and over (currently £10.70 and £13.15, respectively). Some practices are slack about registering new patients, and if the delay in sending the medical card or FP1 takes it past the quarterly counting day, the quarter's capitation fee will be lost. Practice managers can make sure that new arrivals register at their first visit, by filling in an FP1 there and then, if they do not have a medical card with them. People who go abroad for short periods may be removed from the list. An alert clerk will notice the entry in the weekly list of removals of patients from the list (FP22A) and take appropriate action. Changes of address should be notified promptly to the FPC, as a letter to the patient from the FPC returned as 'gone away' results in their removal from the list after due notice.

Item of service fees

These fees come in three categories:

1. To recognize special skills and interests of doctors, or to leave them free to opt out, such as maternity work or contraception.
The patient is able to choose a doctor for these services, other than the doctor with whom they are registered. Such fees are for:
    maternity services;
    contraceptive services;
    fitting of an intrauterine device.
2. To remunerate the doctor for work done which is not covered by his terms of service, or for patients not on his list:
    emergency treatment fees;
    immediately necessary treatment fee;
    temporary resident's fee;
    arrest of dental haemorrhage;
    anaesthetic (general) for emergency.
3. As an incentive to doctors, as part of public policy
    vaccination and immunization fees;
    cervical cytology test fee;
    night visit fees.

Item of service fees give the doctors considerable freedom to decide how they wish to practice. They may or may not provide maternity and contraceptive, and cervical screening services, they can give a complete immunization programme, and they can do many or few night visits. These choices are reflected in the remuneration received. It is unlikely that doctors decide to do any of these things just for the money. But having decided as a policy which services they wish to undertake, it is then up to the practice manager to see that the service runs smoothly (as described in Chapter 10 and Appendices A and C), and that fees are claimed properly.

Left to himself, the doctor will often not bother with the paperwork, so a simple system needs to be designed, so that fees are claimed for all work actually done. Examples of lost fees to which the practice manager might give attention are:

(1) contraceptive services, not claimed annually on time;
(2) miscarriages not claimed;
(3) emergency treatment at night and weekends, not claimed;
(4) night visits not claimed;
(5) immunizations not claimed;
(6) reminders not sent.

It is not difficult to set up a checking system to close the loopholes through which money, legitimately earned, runs to waste.

Other allowances and payments

A number of other fees and allowances are payable by the FPC. These include:

(1) postgraduate training allowance;
(2) training grant;
(3) trainees' salary and allowances for car, London weighting, etc. †
(4) retainer scheme payments for married women;
(5) initial practice allowances for practising in seriously under-doctored area;
(6) rural practice payments;
(7) dispensing payments;
(8) sickness payments;
(9) prolonged study-leave payments and locum allowance;
(10) fees for reports to RMO, etc.;
(11) expenses of attendance at postgraduate meetings (Section 63).

The practice manager needs to be aware of these fees. Payment of trainee allowances has been mentioned in Chapter 4. Rural practice payments and dispensing payments can be an important source of income. They are described more fully in *The business of general practice*, quoted in the section on 'Income tax'. All general practitioners can claim for items personally administered such

† Removal and telephone expenses are paid direct to trainee.

as drug injections, vaccines, pessaries, intrauterine devices (see paragraph 44.13 of the 'Red Book').

NHS revenue separate from the FPC

Doctors may be paid for sessional work for hospitals or social services, community hospital work, lectures to health authority staff, and so on. These fees will be paid by the health authority, and national insurance, tax, and superannuation may be deducted. A careful record of all these payments and deductions must be kept. The practice accountant may be able to arrange with the paying authority and the inland revenue for tax not to be deducted.

Non-NHS revenue

GPs receive income from a wide variety of sources. This is a measure of the breadth of the doctor's role in the community. Such fees are usually paid at rates agreed with the British Medical Association, so an up-to-date schedule of fees is needed. Members of the BMA can find this in their handbook, and regular supplements are available on request. An abbreviated version is printed in *Medeconomics* and *Pulse*. The *BMA handbook* has a useful list of certificates and service for which a charge may *not* be made. Fees charged to private patients are subject to negotiation between doctor and patient, and there are no recommended levels. However, the fees paid by Government bodies for visiting a doctor, or for a home visit, may be used as a guideline. It is important that the practice has clear policies about levels of fees and exemptions (e.g. for pensioners, nurses, doctors, dentists, etc.).

The practice manager's aim of maximizing revenue is not achieved by goading doctors and staff to greater efforts, but by ensuring that fees earned are claimed and paid; and streamlining those services in pursuance of public policy where extra revenue is available. She can also gather information about the profitability of various parts of the work so that the partners can take more rational decisions about policy. This is considered further under 'Financial management', as is keeping accounts of revenue.

If non-NHS fees exceed 10 per cent of the practice revenue, an adjustment is made in the re-imbursement for rent and rates, and for ancillary staff.

If the practice revenue can be kept buoyant, then expenditure on services to patients will be less restricted. This is considered in the next section.

EXPENDITURE

Practice expenses are complicated, and careful records must be kept. Some expenditure (e.g. rent, rates, and staff national insurance) attract 100 per cent re-imbursement; other payments (e.g. to ancillary staff) attract 70 per cent re-imbursement of wages, salaries, and training costs. Some practice expenses are common to all the partners; others (like cars and professional subscriptions) reflect the partner's individual preferences. All expenses which are wholly and exclusively incurred in the practice should be allowable for relief from income tax. These allowances are subject to negotiation between the practice accountant and the tax inspector. A qualified accountant may be consulted, who is familiar with the best way of treating the local tax inspector.

Accounts will need to be kept separately for general practice expenses, and personal expenses. The practice manager would normally be responsible for the former, while the individual partner and the accountant might deal with the latter. Further discussion of income tax is deferred until the section on 'Income tax'.

The main categories of capital and revenue expenditure

These are listed below (for more detail see the section on 'Financial Management' – accounts:

(1) premises (capital costs, maintenance, rent and rates, etc.);
(2) staff pay-roll (non-medical; medical, e.g. locums);
(3) postage, stationery, telephones;
(4) equipment (purchase or leasing) and library;
(5) bank interest and charges;
(6) accountancy and legal fees;
(7) superannuation.

Personal practices expenses

These might include the following, though with agreement, some could be met by the practice:

(1) superannuation (deducted through practice);
(2) car expenses, including depreciation;
(3) professional subscriptions;
(4) refresher courses, books, journals;
(5) household expenses in connection with the practice, e.g use of room as study, or for seeing patients;
(6) telephone expenses, and someone to answer the telephone.

From the information supplied by the practice and partners the accountant will prepare a balance sheet, and revenue (profit and loss) accounts for submission to the Inland Revenue. The practice manager will also need to give much more detailed information to the partners to help them make decisions about expenditure.

The dilemma has been mentioned whereby doctors who pay out little in patient services may have a higher net income – though the taxman takes his slice. How does the practice manager help to guide the partners to an equitable compromise? A simple calculation from the annual practice accounts will show the net and gross practice income, and these figures can be compared with the national averages shown in, for example, *Medeconomics*, so that partners can see how they compare with the average, both for net income before tax, and in the percentage of practice expenses compared with the national average of about 33 per cent. For accuracy, personal practice expenses will have to be included in the sum. Practices which pride themselves on their service to patients often have expenses well above the average, but offset these expenses by a higher-than-average gross practice income. About half the practices have to be above the average line, so an equitable balance must be agreed and monitored from year to year. If, however, the main aim of the partners is to maximize their net income, then the practice manager will have to work harder to justify expenditure and maximize revenue.

There are different ways of scrutinizing expenditure:

net cost;
opportunity cost;
marginal cost;
cost-effectiveness.

Net cost

An example to illustrate this is the employment of a full-time practice nurse (or treatment-room sister):

Salary per annum (Grade G)		£12 975
Less re-imbursement at 70 per cent	£9082	
Net cost before tax		£ 3893
Less tax at 40 per cent	£1557	
Net cost		£ 2336

In a practice of four partners, each would be poorer by £584 per annum. But the nurse could be expected to generate revenue, and her pre-tax net cost of £3893 would be covered by her doing 200 cervical smears and 550 immunizations at higher rate. Pritchard (1981) quotes a treatment room sister as doing about 200 smears and 500 immunizations per annum, which alone would nearly cover the cost of employing her, if they all attracted a fee. Similarly, if a new partner is engaged, a substantial proportion of his or her share of the profits is offset by an increase in allowances.

Opportunity cost

The same treatment-room sister quoted above did, in addition, over 8000 other tasks in the year – many of which would otherwise be done by the doctor (e.g. suturing, dressings, blood taking, ear syringing, injections). This gives the doctor the opportunity to spend the time freed in other ways. It could be in spending more time with patients, in earning money, or in playing golf. He is free to choose.

So in considering how to spend money, one must consider the opportunity it provides to do things differently, and compare one option with the opportunities for benefit by spending the money in other ways. A topical national example is whether to spend £½ million on heart transplants, or on prevention of heart disease. By collecting data and doing the sums, one can come nearer to the decision, but usually value judgements must be made about the 'best-buy'.

Marginal cost

This is a useful concept when there is a going concern, and the plan is to add something on to it.

A simple example is the practice photocopier. If, at the current rate of use, the copies work out at 4p each, would an extra 500 copies a month cost £20? The answer is no. Certain costs like leasing and maintenance are fixed. The extra copies would attract an additional 'copy charge', charged by the leasing company, plus the cost of paper. The total might be 1.75p or £8.75. This does not take into account the additional labour cost of working the machine. But would extra hours be worked, or money lost in other ways? If not, then no labour charge need be added. The practice may not have a photocopier, but wishes to run off some leaflets for patients. If the local Health Authority would not do it free (as health education), at least a marginal cost might be negotiated which would be fair for all.

Cost-effectiveness

In order to compare the different options for spending money, measures of outcome related to that expenditure are needed. Very rarely can one say 'if I spend a sum of money on a particular project, then so many patients will benefit to such-and-such an extent'. This lack of a complete picture, should not deter the practice manager from weighing up the likely benefits from various plans which she and the partners have in mind.

Some plans may not benefit patients directly, but benefit the staff in terms of efficiency and morale. These should not be underrated. If we do not have satisfactory measures of the outcome of health care, we can next think of the process of giving care. Three important determinants are:

(1) the skill of the staff members involved;
(2) their morale and dedication;
(3) the efficiency of the teamwork and communication.

Without accurate measures, it is a good assumption that money spent on training, on motivation and morale raising, and on communication and team-building is money well spent.

When undertaking cervical screening or child immunization, all goes smoothly at first, but after, say 50 per cent have been done, the cost begins to rise. One is dealing with more-reluctant patients with perhaps greater difficulty of access. After a certain point of flagging notes and sending reminders, the take-up slows down or stops. At what point is the decision made to accept the situation? The cost of having the last 5 per cent of children immunized, or the last 30 per cent of women screened, may not be worth the effort. With experience of such programmes, the plans may be modified to achieve a realistic aim of 95 per cent of children being immunized, and a 70 per cent take-up of cervical screening.

INCOME TAX

Accountancy, like medicine, is a highly specialized profession. An accountant skilled in tax, and with some knowledge of general-practice finance, will be needed. This section cannot provide a comprehensive tax guide, but only some hints for the practice manager and partners in playing their very important part in the process. The aim is not to evade paying income tax, but to pay no more than is legal and necessary. Many practices forgo money by not claiming expenses against tax, just as they fail to claim revenue to which they are entitled.

Having chosen an accountant, then the practice accounts must be presented in an acceptable form. The accountant will advise particularly on the allowances which can be claimed for motoring expenses, for household expenses when patients are seen at home, or when practice work is done at home. Some inspectors will accept a formula; others will expect mileage to be logged for a test period. All allowances claimed should be based on fact.

The relationship between the practice, the accountant, and the inspector must be based on mutual trust. It is not a good policy to try to outsmart him; this may jeopardize future relationships.

The practice manager's role is to ensure that accurate accounts are produced, which include *all* expenditure properly incurred by the practice. If the partners pay out of their wallets, and no note is taken or receipt sought, then they will be the losers. The practice manager, in all but the smallest practices, will probably have the help of a wages-clerk/secretary, who will do the payroll (PAYE) and keep the various accounts. It is an advantage if the accounts for the partnership are presented to the accountant in as finished a form as possible, otherwise his fee may be large. Paying audit-clerks and chasing up missing data may add several hundred pounds to the accountant's bill; whereas a clerk/secretary in the practice can have 70 per cent re-imbursement of her salary, provided that she meets the qualifying conditions on the 'Red Book'. It is helpful if one partner, or the practice manager (or both), takes a particular interest in tax matters, and acts as the link with the accountant.

The Inspector of Taxes, having received the accounts, will work out an assessment of the partnership's (not the individual doctors') liability to tax. The accountant will work out the individual partner's shares, but the practice is liable for the tax. The usual payment dates are 1 July and 1 January. Delay in payment may result in interest being charged. If the amount of tax claimed is subject to appeal, the accountant will advise how much to pay on account.

Wage and salary earners are taxed at source by PAYE under Schedule E, whereas partners in a business pay on the profits of the business as shown in the certified accounts, under the Schedule D regulations. It is too complicated a story to describe here. The reader is advised to refer to the sources of information listed at the end of this chapter.

CAPITAL

Most of this chapter has referred to revenue and expenditure – the 'profit and loss' part of the accounts. Buildings, equipment, and cars have been mentioned; they come into a different category, as fixed assets on which the capital value of the practice is assessed. This capital is jointly owned by the partners, usually in shares related to their share in the practice. So a well-established practice of four partners might have equal (quarter) shares, but a new partner might start with a smaller share.

The building (if owned by the practice), the equipment, and the cars will all depreciate due to wear and tear, though the value of the building may increase with inflation of property values. The accountant can use a formula to assess the value from year to year which is accurate enough. However, if a partner leaves, he will want to withdraw his share at a more exact current value, so a professional valuation of the building and equipment (and drug stocks) may be needed.

A similar stocktaking is required when a new partner joins, or his share changes. It saves trouble if these events take place on the accounting date of the practice, but tax liability must be considered before a date is decided. Cars have a different system of valuation against tax, and a more precise value might have to be put on them if they belong to the practice, or are sold. This is also an area for the accountant's expertise, but the practice manager will have to keep accurate inventories of equipment, with their initial value, and date of purchase. This is important for tax purposes, for changes of partners or shares, and for insurance. Any newly-bought equipment must be entered in the inventory, and a supporting invoice kept for the accountant.

If the book value of the stocks is far below the actual value, then the partnership may get a shock if a true valuation shows a considerable rise in value. This counts as a profit, and is taxed heavily, whereas if the gain in value had been spread over several years, the tax might have been less heavy.

The balance sheet is likely to contain the following headings:

Fixed assets	Buildings..
	Medical and office equipment (listed)................................
Current assets	Stock of drugs and dressing...
	Debtors...
	Cash in hand..
Less	Current liabilities ....

Net assets

Each partner will have a separate capital account to represent his share of the assets, both capital and revenue, less his drawings from the partnership and superannuation. This allows for the fact that partners pay different amounts of tax, so their drawings may not always keep exactly in step.

Financing practice premises

Let us imagine a situation where the partners have decided that they would like new premises. What are the next steps in financing the plan, and in how can the practice manager help?

1. *Obtain a clear brief.* How big a building is needed? Where will it have to be located in relation to the practice area? How soon is it needed? Will it be for sole practice use, or shared with other practices or agencies such as health visitors and social services? These are some of many questions, the answers to which will affect the outcome.

2. *Obtain information.* In addition to the references given in Chapter 14, there are a number of useful publications on financing practice premises which must be studied in detail:

(a) *Statement of fees and allowances* ('Red Book'), paragraph 51.
(b) *The business of general practice.* (3rd edn). General Practitioner/GMSC.
(c) *The general practitioners' year book, Part I,* 1982. Winthrop Laboratories.
(d) Articles in *Medeconomics, General practitioner in practice Supplements,* and *Pulse.*

Advice should be sought at an early stage from:

(a) The Administrator of the Family Practitioner Committee.
(b) The DHSS Regional Medical Officer.
(c) The British Medical Association (for Members).
(d) The Information Resources Centre (RCGP).
(e) The Bureau of Medical Practitioner Affairs (addresses in Appendix F).

3. *Weigh up options.* Upon detailed enquiry it will be found that some options will be excluded (e.g. no NHS capital may be available for Health Centres). The remaining options must be tabulated in detail for presentation to the partners, with the advantages and disadvantages listed and compared. The whole undertaking must be costed, with allowances for re-imbursement. Professional fees, which can be heavy, should be included. It would not be possible to cover the options comprehensively in this short section, but a summary of ways of financing premises is set out in Table 13.1.

Table 13.1 *Financing general practice premises: summary of options available*

Owner	Comments	Method of financing
District Health Authority	Health centre (or Medical centre in hospital campus)	No capital cost to practice. Rent and rates paid by FPC direct to DHA.
Local Authority	Medical centre (or use of council house etc.)	No capital cost to practice. Economic rent † charged, which may exceed notional rent, † but usually re-imbursed by FPC
Developer or Landlord (who may be retired partner)	Buy and lease back, or normal tenancy agreement	Normally no capital cost to practice. Notional rent agreed with FPC in advance (or cost rent † scheme)
General Practice Finance Corporation (GPFC)	Capital cost limited by SFA, Para. 51. Buy and lease back	Cost rent initially then option to transfer to notional rent
Partners	Partners must repay loan, but gain any appreciation in value	Loan from finance house, building society, or GPFC. Cost rent (if new or substantially modified premises), otherwise notional rent. Improvement grant may be available ‡

† Economic rent: rent based on actual cost to local authority; notional rent: rent fixed by District Valuer; cost rent: interest at GPFC rate on actual cost (within certain limits)
‡ Improvement grant regulations are complex. Enquiry should be made of practice accountant and FPC. See 'Red Book', para. 56.

FINANCIAL MANAGEMENT

Keeping accounts

Much has been said already about keeping accounts in relation to capital, revenue, and expenditure. The mechanics will be considered here.

Capital accounts

These must include the inventory of buildings, equipment (medical and non-medical), and securities. Initial value, date of acquisition, and current value will be entered annually on the accounting date, which is decided in discussion with the accountant. There may be advantages in using 30 June rather than 31 March as the date, depending on the circumstances of the practice.

Revenue accounts

These consist of a bank cash book in which all accounts paid in are listed, and if possible the heading described (e.g. private fee, FPC quarterly cheque). The entries should be numbered, and this number should apear on the supporting statement. They must be put in a box file, or treasury-tagged in the same order. Several cheques may be paid in on the same date, and these entries must be checked against the bank statements.

The headings of revenue required for practice management are many, so an analysis book (preferably loose-leaved) will be needed, with 20 or more columns, It is important in cases where there is re-imbursement, in whole or in part, to put in the full gross amount in the revenue and expenditure analysis, not just to 'net it off'. (For example, the rent of a health centre is never actually paid, and is cancelled by the re-imbursement on paper.) The accountant's advice should be sought about the headings and layout of the cash book, and other records.

Detailed analysis of the FPC quarterly statement is useful but this would add unreasonably to the size of the analysis book; one compromise is to use the FPC statement as it stands. The procedure is to photocopy the statements as they come in quarterly, and glue them together so that the heading appears only once, and the columns of figures are in series for the whole year. In this way the quarterly and annual trends can be followed, as shown in outline in Table 13.2.

Table 13.2 *FPC statement of fees and allowances for quarter ending........*

Previous year's total	Item on statement	Quarter 1	2	3	4	Annual total
	Standard capitation fees Elderly capitation fees . . . . Temporary resident fees Night visit fees Cervical cytology Immunization Contraceptive services					
	TOTAL					

By using this method the partners and staff can have a detailed analysis of trends, and the practice accounts can be simplified by reducing the number of headings from the proforma to about three.

e.g. capitation fees and allowances;
item of service fees;
seniority payments, etc.

The proforma of deduction could be treated in a similar way

e.g. superannuation;
use of health centre/or loan repayments.

Ancillary staff re-imbursements appear on a separate proforma, and they must be entered in the accounts as well as the gross staff pay, rather than only entering the difference, or net cost. It is helpful to have separate entries for the practice nurse's salary and training, and re-imbursement to balance against the item of service payments which she helps to earn for the practice.

Expenditure accounts.

These can be kept in the same cash-analysis book as the bank cash book. The headings of the analysis should be agreed with the accountant and the partners. Payments by cheque should be with the bank statements.

The payroll

The staff payroll is a standing operation which presents no special problems. Information is needed from the payroll account in order to complete the quarterly re-imbursement forms ANC 2 and 3, so it is helpful to use the payroll stationery produced specially for this purpose by Lloyd-Hamol Ltd. †

Practices employing many staff can obtain re-imbursement for up to a total of two full-time employees (38 hours per week) or the equivalent in part-time staff. If the practice is approaching or exceeds the limit, careful records of hours will have to be kept. An extra allowance is made for locums or additional hours worked to cover holiday, sickness, and training courses. Full details must be stated, particularly if the hours exceed the limit of 76 per partner per week. The 'Red Book' must be studied in great detail to obtain the full re-imbursement to which the practice is entitled. For further information see *Croner's reference book for self-employed* (reference at end of chapter).

Petty cash

The practice manager, by keeping a close eye on the petty cash account, will be able to ensure that no money is wasted, and full tax relief can be claimed where appropriate. Invoices or receipts should be kept to cover all expenditure if possible, in order to satisfy the accountant and tax inspector. If the practice manager is able to sign small cheques, then less reliance needs to be placed on the petty cash account, and so less cash needs to be kept in the building. It is wise to keep all ledgers and account books, as well as cash, in a fire-proof safe, securely fixed to the floor.

The practice manager and partners must have a good working relationship with the practice accountant, as has already been stressed. Reducing the amount of work he and his clerks have to do, will allow him to focus his attention where it is really needed, namely to minimizing the liability to tax. It will also minimize his fee.

How to help the practice accountant

1. Keep neat and accurate cash-analysis book of income and expenditure.
2. Ensure that figures add up and balances are correct, and correspond with bank statements.
3. Keep file of documents about money paid in, e.g. FPC statements.
4. Keep invoices of money paid out in date order.

† Clerk Green, Batley, West Yorkshire.

5. Have full practice accounts ready for the accountant as soon as possible after the end of the tax year.

6. Send all original documents to accountant, i.e.

cheque counterfoils;

bank statements and cash-analysis book;

invoices of money paid out and received;

petty cash book, and any other accounts, wages book;

FPC invoices, superannuation, rent and wages re-imbursements, etc.;

list of equipment and book value.

7. Where the account books may be needed before the accountant has returned them, a photocopy should be taken.

8. Answer accountant's queries promptly and in writing.

9. Inform accountant of impending changes in practice, i.e. new partners, partnership shares, purchase of cars, equipment, etc.

10. Communicate with the Inland Revenue regarding partnership tax matters only through the accountant.

Information for management and planning

The practice manager will scrutinize the accounts closely to see where the money comes from and where it goes, to ensure that there is no waste. The accounts cannot be detailed enough to cover all possible enquiries, so from time to time spot checks or special surveys can be done to answer specific questions, or to fill in the detailed cost of possible new ideas, such as a different telephone system or extra staff. The options open to a practice to change things are not as wide as in a commercial business or industry which constantly has to review marketing and profitability and has clear outcome measures, such as profits. A detailed management information system is probably not yet feasible at practice level – except perhaps into the cost-effectiveness of prescribing.

Information for district planning of primary health care services is still sadly lacking. There are figures of where the money goes (from FPCs and Health Authorities) but virtually no linkage between money spent and effectiveness of patient care. The NHS thinks, or hopes, it is getting good value for money in primary health care, but evidence is scanty. Until hard evidence of outcomes of primary health care are available, requests for more resources may fall on deaf ears. Too much pre-occupation with money diverts the doctors from their main role, so it is important for the practice manager to have the financial management of the practice under firm control. She will need detailed knowledge, so that the partners can delegate most of the money worries to her, with confidence. However, this does not mean that the partners lose financial control.

Financial control

Control of the financial element of an organization cannot be divorced from the system as a whole, and particularly from its planning and policy-making. If the practice wants to move in a particular direction, but the financial control prevents it, the result will be frustration. Financial control is inseparable from the consideration of policies, priorities, and decision-making. These topics crop up in several chapters in this book, and are not repeated here. However, the dilemma facing general practitioners must be re-stated.

High-quality service to patients costs money and does not usually generate extra revenue, so the more conscientious doctors will be poorer, unless they are extra-smart in generating more revenue.

Major decisions on spending are usually taken in a partners' meeting, and often there is sharp division of opinion between the innovators and the laissez-faire faction. Even a majority decision may not be the answer if it means spending everyone's share of the practice income. So laissez-faire is more likely to prevail. In addition, some partners may have much heavier financial commitments, such as school fees, and look twice at every penny. It is difficult to escape from this trap in the case of major expenditure, but if every minor expense is vetoed, then management of the practice can become very inefficient. One answer is for the practice manager to have a free hand with the petty cash (subject to a monthly cash limit) and to have a budget for maintenance, library books, and so on, which she can spend up to the budget limit. The expenditure will still be open to scrutiny by the partners, but she will not need to go cap-in-hand every time she needs to make minor purchases.

Budgets do not play a major part in general practice finances, as it is not that sort of business, but some budgets are helpful as described above. In any case, the expenditure will be scrutinized after the event.

Who signs the cheques? In some practices the manager signs all the cheques, including the partners' monthly payments. In others two signatures are needed on each cheque, one of which may be the practice manager's. In a large practice there are many cheques to sign. So a system, such as a separate imprest account for the practice manager will save the doctors' time, and is worth considering.

COMPUTERIZATION OF ACCOUNTS

Before computerizing general practice finance, the questions posed in Chapter 12 must be asked, in particular:

   (1) what do we want to do?
   (2) will a computer do it better?
   (3) is it worth the cost and trouble?

As with medical records, there are several stages of complexity and cost. For example:

   (1) payroll;
   (2) item of service payments;
   (3) revenue and expenditure accounts;
   (4) complete practice accounts;
   (5) liability to income tax.

Computerizing the payroll

This is a relatively straightforward task, for which many ready-to-use programs can be bought, and only a small microcomputer is needed. As mentioned under payroll, some modification is needed to suit the claims for re-imbursement, but this should not present a problem. It is quite a good exercise in the use of a computer for the practice to undertake, before expanding into other fields. Manual records must still be kept, but the computer can work out the PAYE and do all the sums, with a print-out for the records and an individual pay-slip for the employee. It would save the clerk some time, but re-training in the use of the computer might be needed.

Seventy per cent of the clerk's salary is re-imbursed, and a minimum of 5 hours a week is needed to qualify for re-imbursement, so cash savings are unlikely, though accountant's fees might be less. The service will be as efficient as the wages-clerk who runs it, so an increase in accuracy is unlikely in a small organization. The conclusion might well be that a computer just to do the payroll of a small organization would not pay, but as part of a larger, or developing system it might be justified. If the practice does not have a computer, a bank or bureau may do the payroll on their computer for a fee.

Item of service payments

Filling in a multiplicity of different forms for different purposes, costing them, and checking that the FPC has made payment, is a very laborious process. A computer could make it much easier, but not if the current forms still have to be filled in as well. A standard claim form which could be filled in on the computer keyboard, with suitable prompts to remind the operator, would be a start. Computer-compatible stationery (as for FP10s) would be necessary. Then the one entry could put in the claim, cost it, and enter it into an account under the appropriate heading, generate a record for the notes, and diary the date the next claim is due. Some FPCs will accept computer-printed claim forms. Their co-operation should be sought at an early stage.

Revenue and expenditure accounts

The computer is not as good as a clear analysis-book at recording and displaying accounts. What it can do is to add up and process the information more easily. The written records may still be needed, both in order to generate the computer record and in case of accidental loss of the computer memory, but need not be kept in such detail.

Many accountants now have computers, and can save much time and effort in processing the data, and assessing tax liability. Looking well into the future, the practice accounts could be handled by a computer, and stored on floppy disk which is then sent to the accountant annually to feed into his machine. This would save duplication of the difficult bottleneck of computerization – namely data-input.

Complete practice accounts

Theoretically, the whole accounting process could be done on a practice computer. A decision would depend on the size of the organization, and ease of data input. A discussion with the practice accountant would resolve the issue. Success would depend on him being an experienced computer-user. A computerized accounting system would allow more processing of financial data than occurs at present, which could produce better information for decision-making than is available, or even contemplated now.

Liability to income tax

This subject is in the sphere of the accountant, and beyond the scope of this book.

Imposition of cash limits on FPC expenditure

To date (1988) Family Practitioner Committees have been able to meet all calls for expenditure justified by the 'Red Book' and Departmental guidelines. This may all change if cash limits are imposed on FPC expenditure. The limits may well fall on staff and building costs and so inhibit those practices that are trying to deliver a better service.

SOURCES OF INFORMATION ABOUT PRACTICE FINANCE

The business of general practice (3rd edn) (1983/4). Prepared by *General Practitioner* and *Medeconomics* for the General Medical Services Committee. (Obtainable from BMA.)
Hambro tax guide (published annually). Oyez-Longman, London.
Daily Mail income tax guide (ed. R. Tingley). Harmsworth Publications. Published annually in the month or two following the Budget (i.e. about June).
General Practitioner. In *Practice Supplements.*
Pocket Guide to the Red Book (1988/9).
Money Pulse (Regular articles on finance.)
Medeconomics (Regular articles on finance.)
Croner's reference book for the self-employed and smaller business. Croner Publications, 173 Kingston Road, New Malden, Surrey.

Section C

'Things'

14 The building

In the days before the National Health Service (pre-1948) it was commonly accepted that a general practitioner would set aside a room in his own home where he could see his patients. Half the doctors in the country worked completely on their own. Purpose-built health centres were almost unknown.

The Doctors' Charter of 1966 had a tremendous impact on primary medical care. The 100 per cent refund of rent (as assessed by the district valuer), and rates of surgery premises, and 70 per cent refund of staff salaries, has encouraged doctors to improve their premises or move to a health centre.

It is a condition of the *Statement of fees and allowances* that the doctor, whilst contracting to look after the medical care of his patients, will provide adequate consulting and waiting facilities. General practitioner premises vary from two small rooms to the very large purpose-built centres. Purpose-built premises do not necessarily equal good medical practice, but with community care now receiving greater emphasis, good practice will need good premises.

MAINTENANCE

Many doctors will have invested considerable sums of money in their premises, either directly, or by a capital share when joining an existing partnership. They will expect their investment (the building) to be looked after. Most practice managers will be given the task of organizing and supervising schedules for cleaning and maintenance. In publicly owned buildings such as health centres this will be the administrator's responsibility. She will be accountable to the Health Authority, not the practice, but her aim will be similar – an efficient and acceptable service to patients and staff.

The daily routine

A reliable, responsible cleaner who can work unsupervised is a tremendous asset to the practice. He or she should be employed in a serious, efficient manner and, as with other members of staff, given a clear job description covering all her duties. The surgery, like any other building accessible to the general public and open for possibly ten hours a day will, by closing time, look messy.

Routine cleaning of furniture, upholstery, carpets, other flooring, toilets, sinks light fittings, etc. can be written down as a work procedure. Cleaning a large practice will be expensive, but there is no short cut. The practice manager will have to ensure that broken and faulty equipment (vacuum cleaner, step ladders, etc.) is reported immediately, in order that a replacement can be arranged. A system for maintaining adequate supplies of soap, towels, toiletries, and cleaning materials should be explained and understood by the cleaning staff. Because of the necessity to clean the premises during unsocial hours, it could prove difficult to find a reliable person and the practice manager may find it more satisfactory to summon the assistance of a firm of contract cleaners. One can simply turn to 'Yellow Pages' (office cleaning, carpet and upholstery cleaners, window cleaners) and make enquiries to obtain the most suitable service at a budget price. Firms will be able to quote a price (which will include the use of their equipment). It is wise to seek and take up references before signing a contract.

The doctor may pay the cleaner whatever is mutually agreeable, but it is fair to check with the supervisor of the domestic services at a local hospital or college who will be able to quote the current rate per hour for domestic services.

There is a vast range of cleaning materials, domestic and industrial equipment on the market; a market that is constantly being updated and improved. The practice manager is not expected to keep pace with the science of cleaning, but will be expected to be reasonably knowledgeable and at least have a point of contact with the commercial trade, or with the domestic supervisor or supplies officer of the local Health Authority.

The weekly routine

Waste collection

A twice weekly local collection will cope with the normal non-confidential, non-dangerous waste, but special arrangements may have to be made for syringes, needles, and confidential papers. A contractor will collect such material at a charge rate per sack, but in many cases the general practitioner is too small a client for a firm to be interested and the practice would be better served by a special arrangement with the city or district refuse collection service. Some cities have special days on which confidential or dangerous material can be taken personally to an incinerator. There is usually a small charge for this facility.

Towels

Laundering of hand towels may be a specific duty of the cleaner, or towels can be laundered and supplied on a weekly basis by a professional firm. Paper towels are more convenient. Hot air hand-driers have the disadvantage of being noisy.

Mats

Some professional firms can also provide various floor mats for use in heavy-duty areas; mats that are specifically treated to take as much dirt as possible from shoes. These mats are lifted and replaced with clean ones at regular intervals. The charges are reasonable, and over a particularly bad winter of snow and slush, can prove almost essential.

Monthly routine

Window cleaning

Window cleaning once a month would suffice under normal circumstances. Window cleaning contractors, fully licensed and insured are readily available, but employing a local 'handyman' would have the advantage of allowing the practice manager to set a time for window cleaning that would be most suitable to the practice.

Gardening

Once more, 'Yellow Pages' will indicate local professional contractors, but for the smaller garden, the neighbourhood will almost certainly hold a garden enthusiast who would be delighted to undertake a small part-time job.

Spring cleaning (or occasional cleaning)

Carpets

There are specialist firms who will visit the practice and advise on the best methods of cleaning carpets. A list of recommended companies can be obtained from their association.† Alternatively, names can be found in 'Yellow Pages', or recommended by the local Health Authority.

Curtain cleaning

Surgery curtains should preferably be made of fireproof and easily laundered fabric, i.e. cotton, which will stand up to repeated washing and continue to look fresh. The cleaner may undertake some overtime work and launder the curtains. Alternatively, curtains may be dry cleaned. Reproofing of curtains against fire may be necessary.

Regular inspection

Practice premises, regardless of their size, will take a battering. All members of staff should be encouraged to report problems and defects as soon as they are noticed. Detecting faults early and taking action can save substantial bills later. By taking a note of the necessary repairs, painting, and other items of general maintenance, the practice manager will be able to pinpoint areas of priority. It is sensible to organize redecoration on rotational annual basis, rather than be faced with an enormous practice facelift after several years. The practice manager will at this point be overwhelmed at the expectation of her knowledge, but it will be reassuring to note that in this area of domestic science it is perhaps more important to know who to call on rather than how to do it.

† The Carpet Cleaners Association, 299–301 Ballards Lane, London NW

SECURITY

No statistics exist either on the incidence or cost of damage to general practitioner surgeries. General statistics, however, show that this type of crime against premises is on the increase. Surgery premises are obvious targets for burglars and drug addicts, and it is encouraging to note that doctors are taking advantage of the recent extension to the 'Red Book' improvement-grant regulations, which now include fitting security systems. It is important to obtain expert advice. The police crime-prevention officers are acutely aware of the difficulties that exist when premises are left unattended. The Crime Prevention Officer has undergone special training for his profession; his advice is free.

The practice manager and the doctor might be perplexed by the diversity both of quality and cost of alarm systems. The Crime Prevention Officer will indicate an appropriate type of security system. He may also provide a list of suppliers approved by the police. Most companies are members of the National Supervisory Council for Intruder Alarms.

The FPC must be informed before any firm is engaged, since a grant cannot be awarded *after* the work has commenced. The FPC will require three estimates and will generally award the grant on the lowest. Provided the cost is above £500 the FPC will pay one third of it. Paragraph 56 of the *Statement of fees and allowances* states that it will be necessary to call in the Regional Medical Officer if the work exceeds £2500, but the installation of a security system is unlikely to cost as much as this. Security does not mean that the only answer to the problem is a sophisticated, modern, electronic alarm system. The practice manager will have to question 'what needs to be secured?' One room, a dispensary, the whole building? The police will also favour physical deterrents, such as grilles, bars, locks, double glazing, and special security doors.

Any general practitioner wishing to improve the physical security of his premises might be confused by the variety of methods available. The library of the Royal College of General Practitioners has a comprehensive checklist on vandal proofing.† Once again the Crime Prevention Officer of the local police will help to select the best methods.

DESIGN OF NEW BUILDINGS

By far the most frequently mentioned 'tools for teamwork' are the premises from which teams work. Problems raised generally come into two categories, lack of space and poor design, the former more often raised in respect of privately provided premises, the latter in relation to health centres. A recent report (DHSS 1981*a*) details problems relating to both inadequate space and poor design, and recommends that:

† Upjohn Travelling Fellowship (1980/81).
   Is vandal proofing possible? G. Dean.

1. Eventual users of primary health care premises should be consulted during the initial design stages of the premises and be represented on the project team.

2. All new or adapted practice premises should be of sufficient size to accommodate the members of the team and their anticipated activities.

3. New or adapted premises should be designed, whenever possible, to facilitate informal contact between team members.

4. Any revision of the building note on health centres should take account of the comments in respect of size and design of facilities that should be provided and it should so far as possible be sufficiently broadly based to provide guidance on the design of group practice premises.

Whether you work in a single-handed practice or in a large group, the premises will have an effect on your work. Not all GPs have the opportunity to work from health centres, and equally important, not all GPs wish to. Doctors are encouraged to improve their practice premises but building, even at its most modest level, is expensive. Few health centres are being built now, but there is a great deal of activity and development of purpose-built premises, notably under the cost rent scheme. Details of this and other methods of financing premises are discussed briefly in Chapter 13. For more detail, the reader is referred to *The business of general practice* (1983/4) published by *General Practitioner* for the General Medical Services Committee, or *Medeconomics*.

To be involved in the design of a new building, at whatever level, is a stimulating experience. Each practice has its own aims, constraints, and circumstances which the design must take into account. Much has been written on the design of new buildings, which may help the doctor and architect to solve a particular problem, but it is important to remember that no standard formula exists and no one knows better about the needs of the practice than those who work in it. Some sources of information follow:

DHSS Bibliography Series, HB 63 (surgeries), and HB 65 (Health Centres). Obtainable from DHSS, Health Buildings Library, Room 1312, 286 Euston Rd, London, NW1 3DN.
Health centres—a design guide, HMSO.
RCGP – the librarian will supply references.
Information Resources Centre (RCGP).
Design guide for medical GP practice centres, RCGP.
Buildings for General Medical Practice, HMSO.

Let us assume that after thorough deliberation the GPs have decided to build new premises, an experienced architect has been appointed, a site has been acquired, and the briefing has started in earnest. The practice manager has been invited to become a member of the design team. The following areas have been identified where her particular viewpoint would be useful, and are presented as a check-list.

What are you designing for?

(1) Providing exactly the same level of service as before?
(2) Likely changes in list size? Is the practice expanding in area or housing density?
(3) Staffing level – both employed and attached.
(4) Likely changes in record storage – e.g. changing to A4 or computerization.
(5) The trend towards community care.

Design requirements

Reception

This area of first contact for the patient is of critical importance. How the reception of the patient is conducted sets the tone and atmosphere of the practice. It can make or mar the doctor/patient relationship.

The patient's requirements

1. Easy access, especially for those in wheelchairs and disabled people, is essential. (Many designs suggest having reception area placed centrally in the building, but scope for future expansion must be allowed.)
2. An area where private conversations can be held between patient and receptionist is highly desirable.
3. A writing surface for use by patients (signing forms, etc.) is useful.
4. Good lighting.

The receptionist's requirements

1. To be able to see what is going on in the waiting area.
2. A good working surface at a height appropriate for standing or sitting, whichever is required. (Many receptionists actually prefer to stand! Their views can be asked and different counter heights tried out.)
3. Provision for all the appointment books/sheets and other stationery required.
4. Adequate telephone facilities (including a telephone out of view and hearing of patients).
5. An additional work station out of sight from patients.
6. Good lighting. (Receptionists complain that whilst spotlights over the reception desk provide excellent light, they create too much heat for comfort.)
7. A low noise level.

Waiting areas

1. Able to be viewed and supervised from the reception area.
2. Warm but not overheated.
3. Well, but not harshly, lit.
4. Two good sized notice boards, one for health education, the other for information about the practice, or other local information.

5. Chairs or other seating, preferably covered in hard-wearing material that can be washed regularly.

6. A clear and easily understood system for directing patients.

7. Some of the larger premises have a sub-waiting area nearer to the consulting room. This helps to keep noise down, and also has the advantage of avoiding delay if the main waiting area is some distance from the consulting room.

The secretary's office

1. Working surfaces in addition to the typist's desk.
2. Good lighting.
3. Warm but well ventilated.
4. Storage and filing space.
5. A telephone.
6. Power points for equipment (typewriter, audio/dictating machines).
7. Sound deadening surfaces.

The record office

1. Adequate space for the records system to be housed, including space for possible expansion.

2. The height of the filing units should be convenient for staff. (Filing clerks are specially liable to get backache.)

3. Enough circulation space (for filing trolley and staff to pass at ease).

4. Lighting needs especially careful design so that the information on the files can be easily read.

Treatment room

The district nurse or practice nurse will carry out many procedures in the treatment room – injections, dressings, ear syringing, blood sampling, minor surgical procedures, blood pressure checks, routine weighing, consultations, chaperoning.

She will need a room equipped for these tasks.

1. Worktops, which should be easy to clean.
2. Cupboard space, including one lockable cupboard for drugs.
3. A 'clean' sink and a 'dirty sink'.
4. Refrigerator for storage of vaccines, sera, and other injections.
5. Examination couch.
6. Examination light.
7. Sterilizer.
8. Desk or writing surface.
9. Facilities for urine testing.
10. Vinyl flooring which can be cleaned.
11. One, perhaps two, trolleys.

12. Two chairs.
13. Footstool.

Consultation rooms

As a very rough guideline, it is recommended that the minimum size for a doctor's consulting room be 9 m², that is about 12 ft. × 8 ft. If examinations are also carried out in the consulting room, then 12 m² should be calculated as a minimum – roughly 13 ft. × 10 ft.

The consulting room is very personal to the GP, so the design should fit in with his ideas and requirements. There are various standard layouts in the design guides, but it is helpful if the architect or practice manager arranges a mock up in any empty consulting room to ensure that it meets the needs of the GP. If the doctor is left handed, for example, this could necessitate a mirror image of a recognized design. Particular attention will need to be paid to siting of services such as plumbing, power points, examination lights, and telephones. Which way the door is hinged; how the patient comes in, and sits down; and the relationships of desk and chairs must all be considered in detail.

Health visitor's requirements

The health visitor will make much of her contact with people by visiting them in their homes, but she will require a quiet office, interview room, or both.

Her basic requirements are a desk, a telephone, two or three chairs, a filing cabinet, and possibly a fairly large storage cupboard. Health education pamphlets, leaflets, and posters, will require storage, as will health education visual aid equipment.

She will need the use of a larger room for mothercraft classes, antenatal classes, and other group meetings. A practice seminar room could be shared by many users.

Staff room

The staff room can be a multi-purpose room for meetings, discussions, relaxation, and refreshment. It is best sited away from the patient areas, and should have catering facilities nearby and an adjacent staff toilet. There are great advantages in having one room only in which all staff can meet and refresh themselves, rather than separate rooms for doctors, nurses, and other staff.

Corridors

1. Adequate lighting.
2. Non-slip flooring.
3. Clear direction signs.
4. Adequate width for ease of passing, and doors wide enough for wheelchairs.

Toilets

1. Separate toilets should be provided for staff and patients. (One toilet should be accessible to wheelchair users.)

2. Easily cleaned surfaces and flooring.

3. Provision of basin with hot water.

4. Hand drying machines are available that recess completely into the wall, making them more difficult to damage.

5. In premises subject to damage it may be possible to have the entrance to the patients' toilet visible from reception.

6. One toilet with a communicating hatch to the urine-testing area may be useful.

Storage space

Never underestimate the storage needs – most administrators and practice managers will agree that their premises are sadly lacking in storage.

Bulk buying of toilet rolls, cleaning materials, paper towels, strip lights, light bulbs, doctors' notepaper, envelopes, and general office stationery saves money, but requires storage space, which costs money. A place for everything and everything in its place will assist the practice manager in her aim of a smoothly running organization.

Cleaning cupboard or room

The cleaner will work more efficiently and unobtrusively if he has a storage room with a sink.

Refuse

There should be a secure refuse-storage area, inaccessible to dogs, thieves, and drug-addicts. Separate arrangements are needed for 'sharps' and clinical waste (i.e. contaminated dressings), which should be incinerated.

General factors in design

General design factors concerning the practice premises will need to be studied from the start. For example:

1. How is space allocated or shared.

2. Circulation between the various areas of patients and staff.

3. Good communication between the different areas – telephone, intercom, direct voice, transfer of notes, etc.

The physical environment

(1) sound control;

(2) heating;

(3) lighting;

(4) ventilation.

Factors of a psychological nature

There would be little point in providing an efficient building that is physically near perfect without taking special note of the equally important psychological requirements. For example:

(1) colour schemes and textures;
(2) privacy for patients and staff;
(3) rooms with a view;
(4) furnishings and equipment.

Other factors

The architect is the professional who will lead the design team, but he will need to know just as much as you do about the various activities.

A practice manager went as far as requesting the architect to listen and observe in the reception area for a day; it seemed a very good idea. She also encouraged him to visit quite a few health centres and doctors' premises, both good and bad, until the 'feel of general practice' was clear to him!

Apart from the important design and finance elements of new premises, there are, of course the statutory regulations which will cover planning, building regulations, fire, health and safety, and other office regulations. The architect will guide you through these and liaise with authorities, local groups, and neighbours who might be affected by the building.

Designing new premises and seeing them through to completion demands an enormous amount of time. The architect will lead but the practice manager will know the practice inside out, its good and bad points. She should not be afraid to speak out – she has a lot to offer in this field, and will have to endure the mistakes!

Further advice on surgery design and evaluation is available from:

The Bureau of Medical Practitioner Affairs (address in Appendix F);
The Medical Architecture Research Unit, North London Polytechnic, Eden Grove, London, N7; and
The Information Resources Centre, RCGP.

MOVING TO NEW PREMISES

Moving premises, whether on a permanent or temporary basis, will cause serious disruption.

General practice is a 24-hour commitment and cannot be closed for business for three or four days in order to move. If this were possible, moving premises would be much like moving house; employing a firm of professionals and paying heavily for it or undertaking the physical work oneself – getting on with it and feeling exhausted, but very self satisfied, at the end of the move.

The move from one set of premises to the other will probably have to be carried out over the half-day Saturday/Sunday period when the practice will be covered by a duty doctor and the premises are closed to the patients. Given the choice, members of the staff will probably want to supervise their own particular area or department – nurses, the treatment room; receptionists, the reception and records area; doctors, their consulting rooms. With plenty of forethought and planning the pactice manager should be able to ensure an efficient and trouble-free move.

A check-list of suggestions follows. Each practice will have its own special circumstances.

1. Patients notified at an early stage – notices in the waiting area, hand-outs, leaflets from receptionists, and depending on the circumstances of the move, notification to all patients on the list via the FPC.

2. Large clear notices on the door of the 'old' premises.

3. All members of staff and employed staff fully informed.

4. Liaison with the telephone supervisor about arrangements for the transfer period. (Telephone interception if necessary.) Arrangements for insertion in the telephone directory.

5. Practice notepaper and rubber stamps should be amended.

6. Postal services informed.

7. Request all doctors and members of staff to sort out what is absolutely necessary to move, and what can be thrown out!

8. Supervision of all available help into teams to work shifts of a few hours. Everyone working at the one time may be a poor use of resources.

9. If you are lucky, have a handyman on the spot for dismantling filing cabinets, undoing and re-positioning shelves, any small joinery jobs, and removal and replacing of the doctors' plates.

10. Collect as many large boxes and packing cases beforehand as you can lay your hands on, labelled for the rooms in which they will be going.

11. A friend to dispense tea, and keep up the morale!

12. One or two porter-type trolleys are useful: metal filing cabinets are very heavy.

13. Vans and drivers to transport the furniture.

14. Colour-coded or numbered labels on all boxes and furniture, so that they can be directed to the right room in the new premises. Someone must be nominated to ensure that everything goes to the right room first time.

A move will prove exhausting, but when it has been undertaken by the 'all hands on deck' approach and 'it is *our* surgery and we know how *we* want it', it will prove quite an experience, no doubt laced with fun, but above all a further bonding together of the team. If a request has been made to the staff to work over a weekend, despite the fact that time off in lieu has been granted, write and say thank you for a job well done, or have a moving in party when the practice has settled down and is running smoothly and effectively. A 'wine and cheese' type of function is simple to organize and will boost morale.

As a practice manager your identification with the practice may be so great, that inevitably you will take on duties which are not in your job description. If members of staff show the same degree of involvement, thank them.

FIRE RISKS

New building

Building regulations' approval cannot be given unless the proposals are accepted by the fire authorities. The architect will be aware of the regulations and the design will therefore have to conform. Fire doors can have such strong springs on them that frail and elderly people cannot open them. However, they can be fitted with magnetic catches to keep them open, at a cost.

Existing premises

The risks of fire and how to minimize them should be brought to the attention of all users of the doctors' premises. A fire officer from the local fire service will visit your premises on request and advise on precautionary measures. He will provide you with a written report, suggesting additional fire doors, alarms, extinguishers, routes of exit, and fire drill. In larger premises it would be worthwhile to suggest that the Fire Officer meets all staff to explain fire drill. Premises that are old, or have been added on to at various intervals, are particularly vulnerable.

Damage and intrusions on practice premises are bad enough, but do not match the catastrophe of fire damage – particularly when the building and the records are destroyed. A plan to meet this eventuality is outlined in Pritchard (1981). Each practice should work out its fire plan carefully, and precautions should be taken to ensure that the plan itself does not go up in smoke too.

INSURANCE

The risks involved in running and maintaining a surgery are at least the same as those of any other business premises, indeed they may be greater. There is so much choice of insurance cover that it must be scrutinized carefully, or money could be wasted. Insurance cover needs to be specific for surgery premises. In areas where the risk of damage is high, extra premiums may be needed. Full building insurance will include such risks as fire, burglary, theft, damage, water risks, explosion, damage by aircraft, and damage to fixtures and fittings. Contents are insured separately, as are drugs and cash. All-risks insurance may be needed for things taken out of the premises, such as the doctor's bag and car equipment, bleeps, or radio-telephones. Insurance is required by statute for accidental injury to staff, and a certificate to this effect must be displayed on the staff notice board. It is wise also to have cover for accidental injury to members of the public while on practice property. The building should be covered for its full replacement value, which could be double its market value.

Inflation will have to be borne in mind and it is wise to have a policy, and premium, which are index-linked.

HEALTH CENTRES

Most of this chapter has been written for the practice manager employed by general practitioners, and probably working in privately owned premises. Much applies also to health centres, but there are certain specific points worth mentioning.

Health Centres are owned by health authorities, so they have to conform to policies adopted by these authorities, which apply mostly to hospitals. General practitioners have to abide by the rules and pay an agreed sum for maintenance, cleaning, light and heating, and any other services provided, such as reception staff who may be employed by the authority. It pays to keep on good terms with the authority Works Officer, Administrator, and particularly the Treasurer with whom the maintenance charges are negotiated. In small health centres, the practice may employ all the staff and manage the building on behalf of the health authority, for which a small administration charge is made, and added to the bill for services.

Because of capital restrictions and the relative reluctance of GPs to move to health centres, few are being built now, except in such places as new towns. For further information about health centres the reader is referred again to *The business of general practice* (1983/4), and to Beales, J. G. (1978). *Sick health centres,* Pitman Medical, London.

15 Equipment

The surgery building or health centre must be equipped before it can function. Equipment can be fixed, such as cupboards, light fittings, and built-in couches; or it can be moveable, such as desks and chairs. Medical equipment is categorized separately, as are office equipment and electronic equipment.

Fixed equipment

Permanently fixed furniture such as built-in couches, benches, and desks count as part of the building. In health centres they are supplied free and no rent is charged. In privately-owned surgeries they are part of the capital cost against which a loan or buy-and-lease back is arranged. It is usually to the advantage of a practice to have as much equipment built-in as is feasible. However, built-in furniture can limit the flexibility of use or the arrangement of the rooms, so a compromise must be sought. All fixed equipment should be of good quality, as it is less convenient to replace.

Moveable equipment

When moving in to new premises, the widest range of options should be sought. Office equipment and hospital equipment catalogues should be obtained and studied. The Supplies Officer of the Local Health Authority or Board, who is very conscious of quality and prices, should be asked for advice and can often arrange for a practice to share the Authority's bulk-purchasing discount, which can amount to 45 per cent of the quoted retail price. This arrangement can cover all furniture, medical equipment, and items such as typewriters and dictating machines.

MEDICAL EQUIPMENT

Blood pressure machines

These are important items of surgery equipment, and careful choice is needed to ensure quality and ease of maintenance. It may be convenient to have wall-fixed machines near each couch, and a desk model is needed for every consulting room. Some portable models are useful in addition for flexibility when machines are out of service, or for using outside the consulting rooms.

Mercury machines have the advantage of greater accuracy, but must be regularly serviced. A good quality aneroid machine can be very satisfactory, as long as its accuracy is checked regularly against a mercury model. Spilt mercury is a health hazard, so none must be left on the floor after an accidental breakage.

A regular servicing contract is a wise investment.

Weighing machines and height measures

These are needed in every consulting room. To try to economize by sharing is a waste of valuable time.

A steelyard weighing machine is by far the most accurate, but much more expensive than the usual spring model. A compromise is to have a good-quality spring model in every consulting room, and a steelyard model in a central location or in the practice treatment room, where it can be used for (say) antenatal clinics, where greater accuracy is important.

Diagnostic equipment

Diagnostic equipment for the consulting room may be purchased by each partner, according to his preference. However, basic items like auriscopes, opthalmoscopes, patella hammers, and so on, can be bought in bulk, if agreement can be reached on standard models. This makes servicing and replacement cheaper, as well as making it easier for doctors to use consulting rooms other than their own. Some items can be obtained at a discount through journals such as *Pulse* and *Medicine.*

Electrocardiograms (ECG)

These are becoming standard pieces of surgery equipment, but they are expensive. If a practice does not wish to find the capital all at once, they may be leased. It is wise to obtain advice from the local hospital ECG technicians, who will know which machines are reliable. It is an advantage to have a similar make of machine to the smaller portable machines used in the local hospital, so that consultants will be familiar with the format of tracings. In addition, a cheaper service contract may be arranged through the Health Authority if the equipment is similar.

OFFICE EQUIPMENT

Filing arrangements are an essential part of the design of the building, and are considered in Chapter 11. In addition to medical records, the practice manager will need a filing cabinet for administration and easily accessible information. Each partner may want a small filing cabinet in his own consulting room, as well as desk drawers. If there is any problem with choice of filing systems or methods, the Management Services Unit of the Health Authority will usually be ready to advise.

Photocopiers

More than any other piece of office equipment, the photocopier has revolutionized the way people work and communicate. Gone are the days of illegible
carbon copies, ranked in pecking order, so that only the person at the head of
the list could read his copy. For certain, the general practitioner was at the
bottom of the list for hospital summaries! Now all has changed. Carbon paper
need not be used at all, and the circulation of paper is so easy and efficient that
more is produced than anyone can read. Information circulars for patients can
be produced easily, without having to type a master for a duplicator. Information from journal articles can be copied easily and filed away for future reference. There must be a snag, and indeed there is – cost.

There are two main categories of photocopier, plain paper and treated paper.
An example of the former is the Rank Xerox range. The very cheap thermal
copiers, offered to doctors at less than £100, use treated paper. For single
copies or small runs, treated paper is a feasible option, but for longer runs it is
a very expensive way of photocopying. The copies are usually not so crisp, may
fade, and sometimes have a nasty feel and smell. Plain paper copiers have a
higher initial cost (or rental), but this is more than offset by better quality
copies and cheaper paper.

Other factors which have to be taken into account are:

1. Is the copier ready for use immediately, or is there a long warm-up time?
2. What is the speed of copying?
3. Can both sides of the paper be used? This can save paper and postage,
but costs more in labour.
4. Is an efficient maintenance service available?
5. Can a copy be taken from journals and books? (flat-bed facility).
6. How many copies a month are we likely to need?

It is highly unlikely that a practice of less than ten doctors would need
anything approaching 10 000 copies per month. For a three to four doctor
practice, the demand would probably be about 1–2000 per month, depending
on the extent to which they were doing health education and handouts. A
teaching practice might approach the higher figure.

Photocopiers can be bought or leased/rented. Rented machines have in
addition a charge per copy, and a maintenance charge. Calculations could be
done to compare the capital and operating costs of the various copiers. Treated
paper usually costs about 3p per sheet, so is less likely to be competitive. Any
doubts can be easily resolved by requesting the expert advice of the Management
Services Unit of the local health authority.

If the photocopier can be shared with health authority staff, the cost will be
shared also. In a health centre it is likely that a photocopier will be provided by
the authority, and the practice charged a proportion of the cost as part of the
agreed charge. The practice manager will need to ensure that the one supplied is
appropriate to their needs and not unduly expensive. Once again the practice

may benefit by paying discount prices as part of a bulk purchasing deal – for example, photocopying paper would be much cheaper.

Photocopiers can also be used for printing sheets of adhesive labels from a typed master. For commonly used addressees this method saves much time. Overhead projector transparencies for teaching can usually be produced by a photocopier.

Duplicators

These machines have almost been superseded by photocopiers. They require special stencils to be typed, and are usually messy to operate. The copies are not as crisp as photocopies, and the paper is rougher and usually more expensive. Stencils can be cut electronically (e.g. for diagrams) but this is costly, and justified only by a long run. It is probably not worthwhile for a practice to buy a duplicator, but if they have a modern electrically-operated machine, it could be used for runs of 100 or more.

Typewriters

Typewriters can be manually or electrically operated, or electronic. The familiar office or portable machines are usually manually operated. They are obtainable at 'give-away' prices, as the demand for them has fallen. They produce poorer quality typing, and are more laborious to operate than their more modern successors. They have one advantage, apart from price – they can be used in a power cut. It may be a good idea to have one in reserve for when the main machine is being serviced. The health authority Supplies Officer may well have one to 'give away' if approached tactfully.

Electric typewriters

These are much the same as the manual typewriter in construction, but they are driven by an electric motor, which results in better quality of work, greater speed of typing, and less fatigue for the typist. They too are becoming very cheap. They have over 1000 moving parts and so are expensive to manufacture and maintain. A variety of typefaces is available, in 10 or 12 pitch (i.e. letters per inch), or proportional spacing – where the spacing between letters is related to the width of the letter, for example 'w' has more space than 'i'. Proportional spacing gives very high quality typing, resembling a printed page, but is perhaps a luxury. The choice between 10 and 12 pitch rests on legibility. There is no doubt that 10 pitch is more legible, and if handouts are being typed for patients, legibility for those with impaired sight is important. Similarly, carbon ribbon, at slightly greater cost than fabric, gives a crisper result.

Electric typewriters have been entirely superseded by electronic models.

Electronic typewriters

These machines only have about a dozen moving parts, compared with 1500 in the older models. The electronic models have many advantages in terms of speed and convenience. In addition, they can have an extensive memory, so that corrections can be made easily, and a battery of, for example, names and addresses or standard phrases (e.g. notifying appointments or laboratory results) can be stored, and recalled instantly when needed. No special training in their use is required. The only disadvantages are that even these space-age machines break down sometimes, and their initial cost is higher.

There are many makes on the market to choose from. An Olivetti with a small memory storage, for example, is currently priced at £180 and the more elaborate memory typewriter, with a storage capacity of 4000 characters (about three typed pages) currently costs a little over £1000. An enhanced memory of 400 000 characters can be added for an additional £250. The prices quoted (valid in early 1988) include value added tax. Bulk discounts may be available through the health authority. These prices may seem high for a typewriter, but with the likely usage in a practice, the machine could last ten years. The more expensive machine would then cost an extra £100 per annum. But the saving in typist's time should be worth many times this figure.

Once again, the practice manager must obtain the facts and weigh up the options. Advice may be sought as before from the health authority, and the typist should be involved in the choice. The quality of typing reflects the image of the practice.

Word-processors

A word-processor is more than just a memory typewriter. It too has a memory, ranging from 0.25 million characters in the smaller systems to 80 million in the larger systems (in computer language 250 kilobytes, to 80 megabytes or 80 MB). In addition, the word-processor is driven by a more elaborate computer than the memory typewriter, so that it can manipulate the text for purposes of editing, producing statistics, sending standard letters which look like individual ones, and so on.

Some computers, as described in Chapter 12, can be used as word-processors, but they are not always as convenient or efficient as a word-processor designed solely for the purpose.

What does a word-processor consist of? Like a computer it has a typewriter keyboard, with a few additional keys. It has a micro-processor unit, a visual display unit, a printer, and a memory unit usually containing two floppy-disk drives. It is a computer, designed and programmed primarily for one specific purpose – the handling of words and texts – and it needs special programs in order to do many of the other things which computers can do.

Not all practices, at present, would regard a word-processor as essential, but in the future, with the development of screening and prevention programmes, they will become so. For a doctor doing much writing or editorial work they are a necessity:

The cost varies from about £350 for the smaller models, to the more sophisticated ones costing over a thousand pounds. A good quality machine with a daisy-wheel printer more than justifies its extra cost.

Dictating machines

There is now a wide choice of manufacturers and models. It is important that one system be employed throughout the practice, so that the typist has one transcription machine which takes the tapes of all the users. It must have foot controls to leave her hands free. Different users may favour different machines according to the way they work. For example, if they dictate all their letters after the surgery, they may favour a desk model with a hand microphone. If they dictate at odd moments in different places, then the pocket machine is the answer. Different models are available; the smallest is not necessarily the best. All portable models need batteries, and rechargeable batteries with a charger in the office is an option. Practice managers should not forget the secretarial needs of attached nurses. Any increase in their efficiency is of benefit to the practice.

Equipment may be bought or leased. Availability and cost of servicing should be checked before purchasing.

ELECTRONIC EQUIPMENT

Into this category come telephones, bleeps, intercoms, telephone answering machines, and two-way radio. Dictating machines and typewriters have been considered already.

Telephones

Micro-processors have revolutionized telephone systems, and practices considering a change of telephone arrangements should consult the local telephone sales department. They will supply literature and advice, but will not normally do a thorough study of the practice communication system.

It is therefore another task for the practice manager to find out exactly what is needed by each telephone user, and this must all be written down. The major group of telephone users are, of course, patients. Their problems can be discovered by asking a selection of them. (Questionnaires handed out at the hatch for a week will be a start, though this would not include the housebound, who might be questioned via the health visitor.) The telephone manager might agree to monitor the practice lines between 8.30 and 10 a.m. to discover how many calls are made which do not get through – the hidden demand. This might affect the number of lines needed for peak times.

New electronic telephones require much less space than their predecessors and do not need an operator, which can be offset against their higher cost. Their versatility is remarkable. For example, the Herald can operate on 2–10 outside lines serving 4–36 extensions and has an impressive range of functions. An improvement grant may offset the cost of improving the telephone system.

Much time can be saved by push-buttons instead of dialling, and for the central office telephone (or the practice manager's) a callmaker can save much time and frustration – particularly when ringing hospitals which are often engaged. Various types of callmaker are available, which store commonly used telephone numbers, and dial them at the press of a button.

Telephone answering machines

When the surgery is closed, calls must either be switched through to the doctor on duty, or one of the Telecom systems used (e.g. subscriber-controlled transfer, or reference of calls).

An alternative is an answering machine which will give the number of the duty doctor. Some patients find this difficult, and extra coins are needed for call box users, but it is a valuable service. Answering machines which record a message from a patient are less satisfactory, and can be dangerous in an emergency.

Radio pagers

Radio pagers (or bleeps) have established themselves as an essential aid to the duty doctor. When on his round he can be alerted by his bleep going off, so that he rings home or the surgery to get the message. Four different tones are available in one bleep which can distinguish between an urgent and a less urgent summons, or between different callers. The Telecom instrument is very satisfactory and will work in most areas of Great Britain.

Metering cost of calls

A telephone metering device will tell the subscriber how much a telephone call has cost. This is of particular value for long distance or overseas calls which are being charged to a patient or institution.

Intercoms

The telephone will act as an intercom, but sometimes the additional circuit provided by an intercom is useful – for example, to speak to someone else while taking a call. Intercoms are more intrusive than the telephone, but some models can be used when the person taking a call has not got a free hand – as when scrubbed. An intercom to call patients by loudspeaker in the waiting room can be a mixed blessing, particularly if the doctor forgets to switch it off!

Telephone gadgets for the handicapped

The practice manager should be aware of telephone services which are available for handicapped patients, by obtaining the brochure from British Telecom.

Radio-telephones

Radio-telephones (two-way radio) are becoming increasingly popular, particularly for doctors with scattered country practices. The British Telecom system covers the major conurbations, and can link up with the normal telephone network by direct dialling, e.g. from the car. It can be useful for doctors in an emergency, or even if stuck in traffic.

Commercial systems are operated by (for example) Aircall and Securicor which have national coverage, and are portable. Some route calls via the firm's operator, and some link in directly with British Telecom systems, so that any number can be dialled direct. Some link up with a bleep to warn that a call is waiting.

An alternative system is to have a central transmitter and a small number of transmitter/receivers for car or home. This is the sort of system operated by taxi drivers. A central transmitter must be manned, which makes it less suitable for a practice, unless the local hospital or ambulance service will operate it.

All radio-telephone systems are expensive, but are tax-deductible, and may save much time and provide a better service. Patients will often raise money to purchase a radio telephone for 'their' practice.

Section D

Application of management theory

16 Organizations – their varieties and their problems

The whole theme of this book is about people working effectively in organizations to provide a service, which is made up of a multiplicity of tasks.

What are the types of organization in which we work, and to which we have to relate? In what ways does the organization affect the methods of working, and people's inter-relationships and satisfaction? How does an organization relate to a changing society?

There are some of the questions to be considered in this chapter.

WHAT KINDS OF ORGANIZATION?

The hierarchy

In the past, society was organized in a more authoritarian manner, with the boss able to decide on conditions of work, and hire and fire people at will – just as the king or dictator could chop off people's heads at will. This arrangement might have been fine for the boss (or king), but not so good for the employees, who were motivated by the need to obey orders and by fear of the consequences if they did not. In industry, as in government, organizations grew larger so that the boss could not supervise all his workers directly. In response to this there developed a series of levels of authority. Each person had a boss to whom he was accountable, with the ultimate authority residing in the head (or proprietor) of the organization.

Most government bodies and industries still have this hierarchical type of organization on paper, so that some sort of control can be preserved in the implementation of policies, in spending of money, and in matters of discipline (see Fig. 16.1).

Though organizations may be represented in this simplified form, they are unlikely to operate quite like it in practice. The head of the organization may have little real power. He is limited by outside forces, such as legislation, trade unions and markets as well as by many internal factors. For example, many tasks need a group of people to work together, and those people may come from different parts and levels of the organization, and may have many different bosses. These working groups come in various forms, which will be considered in turn.

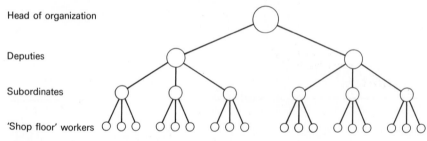

Fig. 16.1. A hierarchical organization. Organizations may have many more levels giving a tall organizational chart, and the lines represent accountability or 'line management'.

Major shortcomings of the hierarchical organization are that it fails to meet people's basic need to be involved in decisions, it does not bring out the best in the work force, it is inflexible, and it tends to treat man as an extension of a machine. The differences between the old style hierarchy and newer organizational structures are summarized in Table 16.1.

Table 16.1. *A comparison of traditional and modern organizational structures*

Old style organization	Newer styles of organization
Technology takes precedence	Human values regarded as important
Man as extension of machine	Man complementary to machine
Man an expendable spare part	Man as a valuable resource to be developed
Tasks broken down into simple narrow skills	Tasks more flexible and requiring broader skills
External supervision and control	Internal self-regulating control
Tall organization chart – autocratic style	Flat organization chart – participative style
Competition, gamesmanship	Collaboration and group cohesion
Concentration on aims of the organization	Individual's and society's needs considered also
Alienation	Commitment
Low risk-taking	Innovation

From: Trist, E. (1981). The evolution of socio-technical systems, in *Perspectives on organizational design and behaviour* (eds. A. Vander Ven and W. Joyce). Wiley Interscience, New York.

Lest we think that this line of thought only applies to large organizations, we can remind ourselves that the NHS, of which general practice is a part, is the largest employer in the United Kingdom and the largest 'hotel and laundry' service in the world. However detached GPs may feel, with their independent contractor status, they employ staff in a hierarchical manner. The attached nurses are part of a separate hierarchy and they have to relate to the NHS organization outside general practice, so need to understand its workings and shortcomings. Because of the defects of hierarchies, other organizational structures and ways of working within a hierarchy have developed.

The task force, project group, or matrix organization

When a particular task needs skills and people from different divisions of a hierarchical organization; from different levels within that organization; or even from outside the organization, then a task force or project team may be set up.

People working in such an organization may have different bosses, be of different status within the organization, and even have a boss outside the organization, or no boss at all. Because of the importance of a task or project, they are encouraged to work together and develop a loyalty to the group, with a corresponding lessening of loyalty to their own boss or even a transfer of it to a boss in a different division. This type of organization is characterized by divided loyalties which inevitably set up strains, yet it can be very successful if the motivation is strong and the potential problems understood. It has worked well in the United States space programme (NASA) and in atomic energy research programmes. Because people have to face two ways, it has been called a matrix organization. The NHS is a giant matrix organization, and we can take an example from a hospital ward to show this in action. Figure 16.2 represents such a unit, where accountability is shown as a vertical line, and co-operation as a horizontal line. The consultant is in a special position as his contract is held by the Regional Medical Officer (except in the case of teaching districts) whereas the other contracts are held at district level. Also, he enjoys a high degree of freedom in making 'clinical' decisions.

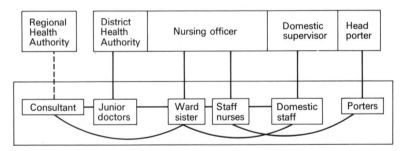

Fig. 16.2. The hospital ward as example of a matrix organization. Vertical lines denote accountability; horizontal and curved lines denote working relationships.

General practice is not a typical matrix organization, but may have certain features of one. The GP has considerable freedom from hierarchical restraints, but has to work closely with people who are subject to these restraints.

The example shown in Fig. 16.3 is of a health centre with several practices in it, which employ their own practice managers and secretarial staff, but rely on

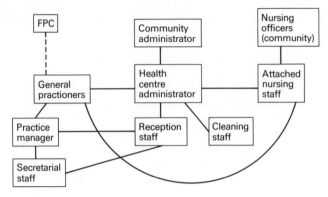

Fig. 16.3. A health centre as an example of a matrix organization. Vertical lines denote accountability; horizontal and curved lines denote co-operation.

reception staff employed by the health authority. The practice nurses have been omitted to save complications. The complexity of such an organization will be apparent and the many crossed lines of accountability and co-operation are not a recipe for easy working relationships. In addition, there are hierarchical elements, and no mention has been made of the team, which is considered later. Matrix organizations are useful where the task involves an input from a number of professionals or technicians, and can be more flexible and responsive to demand. They are said to be more innovative, to conserve resources better, and to favour individual commitment, so they conform to some of the features of the newer style of organization shown in Table 16.1. However, they are not without their problems – one of which is the amount of time required to make them work. Keeping all the channels of co-operation open in the face of demands of line-managers or bosses is hard work, which diverts attention from the task. So can we look for something simpler and smaller?

The autonomous work group or team

In Chapter 5, team working was described and discussed, and two of the four essential characteristics of team work will be repeated here:

1. The members of a team share a common purpose which binds them together and guides their actions.

Whereas a hierarchy or matrix has to work within boundaries largely decided from outside, the team is usually able to set its own boundaries. The tasks are chosen and agreed by the team rather than by individuals, and so they are likely to be more broadly based, and take in the social as well as the technical dimension of the problem. This balancing act will be considered later. So team work should favour an approach which takes into account the individual's problem in the context of the family and society.

4. The effectiveness of the team is related to its capabilities to carry out its work, and its ability to manage itself as an independent group of people.

By definition an autonomous work group must be able to manage its own affairs as far as is feasible. Complete autonomy implies a detachment from outside influences, which could result in autocracy. However, a reasonable level of autonomy is a desirable aim. It can lead to a higher level of self-regulation and of learning from each other. Role flexibility is increased, so that people can give of their best according to their talents, rather than withdraw or feel they have to compete. The increased flexibility can help people to meet domestic, as well as work commitments (e.g. part-time working and flexitime). Job satisfaction is heightened.

For autonomous work groups and teams to succeed, the remainder of the organization must provide appropriate support. In particular, higher management must resist the temptation to 'manage' and control. Rather they should leave well alone, while monitoring to ensure that self-regulation is actually happening.

Designing the organization

Using the framework so far described, we can ask ourselves whether we can improve the design of our organization in terms of structure, process, and outcome. General practitioners have considerable scope for setting up their own organization, as well as improving the function of an existing one – with the practice manager's help. From the experience of other practices, and of other settings, certain conclusions might be drawn, though they will vary according to circumstances. These conclusions are:

1. A small organization is easier to run and more effective than a large organization (i.e. more face-to-face contact).

2. A simple organization produces fewer problems than a complex mixture of hierarchy, matrix, and team.

3. Autonomous work groups have advantages over other systems, but need careful thought and optimum support.

4. Time must be invested in designing the best organization to suit the circumstances.

5. Time must be spent in helping the system function effectively, by attention to internal and external factors.

An example might be for the health centre shown in Fig. 16.3 to streamline its organization, either by having all staff employed by the health authority or, perhaps better, for each practice to function as an autonomous unit, with the function of the health centre administrator limited to looking after the building. Organizational complexities and frustrations are one of the reasons for fewer general practitioners now opting to work in health centres than was the case a few years ago.

Another example might be the practice of four or five partners in an expanding area. Should they go on expanding, or should they decide to limit their area and number of patients, and encourage another practice (or the FPC) to deal with the overflow? The point of trying to ensure that the area covered by attached nursing staff conforms as nearly as possible to the practice area has been considered already.

Investing time in the functioning of the organization is, of course, a major theme of the book.

The network

We have considered the hierarchy, the matrix, and the team, but there is another kind of organization which is highly relevant to general practice – the network. As its name implies it links individuals and organizations together – it crosses boundaries. It often depends on informal ties, whether of family, of common interest, or of friends and neighbours. The linkage may be within an individual, whereby a member of a club or neighbourhood, or a patient of a practice is also a member of a health authority or county council. Networks transmit informal knowledge and consequently power in a community. Their importance should not be underestimated, nor should they be dismissed as improper such as 'the old-boy network'. It is part of reality, and has good and bad characteristics.

A general practice, particularly when it operates in a defined locality, is in a better position to know and use informal networks than almost any other agency. The practice manager is well placed to develop these links, provided her communications with other team members are good. The way in which a patient participation group can develop these networks for the good of the practice and of its patients has been described in Chapter 6.

Whereas the other organizational structures described all operate within boundaries, networks help to make the boundaries less of a barrier and a threat. A practice which is well integrated into the community, and has good links with other community agencies such as social services and housing, will have learnt the lesson about networks.

The organization and society

As mentioned already the trend is away from a purely technical approach to work-tasks towards a more humane approach, which takes into account that workers are people. Similarly, the trend is away from the purely medical model of disease to a wider concept of the causes of ill-health – medical, social, and psychological. The practice organization also has to function as an economic unit. A balance must be maintained between the technical functions of the organization, its social (psychological) functions, and its economics – all this in equilibrium with the world outside the practice. Different practices will produce different balances, but maintaining this balance is an important part of managing the organization. It is a highly complex process, as a glance at Fig. 16.4 will confirm. In looking at this model the practice manager can see how the balance has to be maintained between the three sub-systems, and

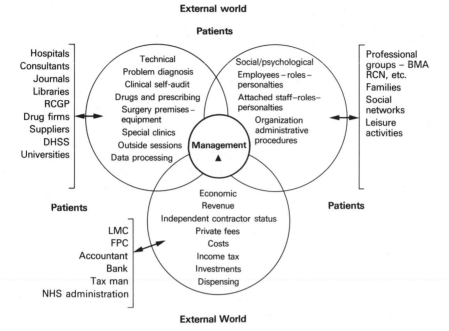

Fig. 16.4. The functions of a practice. A delicate balance.

between the whole system and the external world: particular attention needs to be paid to barriers, which hinder communication; and to the linking mechanisms across the boundaries, which can help effective decision-making.

Fig 16.4 separates the three main functional categories described above. Some possible areas of management interest are included within the circles, but every practice will want to do it differently. In the external world are some of the agencies and people which may be linked to the practice, and of course the patients. This figure may be used as a check-list; or to help one's lateral thinking, by considering who or what has been omitted. There are several limitations to this approach in that it implies that the three functions can be separated; that there are hard boundaries with the outside world; and that it is a steady state, rather than a bustling dynamic process, with people and resources coming in at one end, and health care coming out at the other. The figure represents a snapshot, which perhaps helps one to visualize the milieu in which primary health care operates. How can we draw a model of the process which is nearer to real life?

Primary health care as an 'open system'

Mention has already been made of the concept of the open system, and an attempt will be made here to describe in more detail what this means for primary health care.

Earlier models of organizations do not take into account the complexity of social organizations, or their linkages and interdependence, or the dynamic process which links input into the organization and output, through the process of feedback.

Ideas developed from electrical control systems, from brain function, and from thermodynamics have been found useful in understanding these relationships, and gradually the concept of open systems has developed and been applied to health and social systems.

A system has been defined as 'a dynamic order of parts and processes which interact with one another'. An open system has a less hard and fast boundary, and so can interact more freely with the environment.† What are the basic ingredients of an open system? The critical ones are that it has an input, which is subject to processes which result in a transformation to the output, which is linked again to input by a feedback loop. This system operates in an environment with which it interacts. Figure 16.5 describes a simple system.

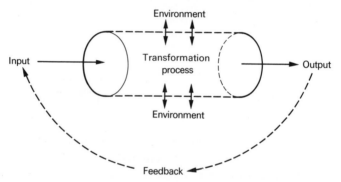

Fig. 16.5. An open system.

Applied to a manufacturing process, it might describe the input of money, manpower, and raw materials into a factory producing soft drinks, with profits as output. The transformation process would involve chemical and industrial processes and control operated by people whose lives are mainly outside the factory. Input would be linked to output by feedback on sales, acceptability, quality control, and trends in popularity of the products. So if too many bottles of one flavour were being produced, the manufacturing process would be modified.

Application to primary health care is more difficult. The input is of money (capital and revenue), manpower other resources, information, and of people demanding or needing health care. The output is better health and satisfied patients. The feedback includes patient satisfaction, measures of health of the population served, and of effective use of resources.

†For further information about systems see: – Open Systems Group (1981). *Systems behaviour*, 3rd Edn. Harper & Row (for Open University) London.

In a stable system there would be an equilibrium, so that improved health lessens demand for care, and releases resources for greater attention to meeting need by case-finding or prevention. If, on the other hand, the health-care process becomes increasingly popular, demand will rise, either until resources run out or feedback measures are introduced to control demand. This would be a more unstable system, and it sounds a bit too real for comfort!

The key to equilibrium is the presence of feedback, so that the relationship of output to input can affect what goes on within the system. Without feedback, the system goes wild. In Fig. 16.5 the feedback loop is shown to run outside the boundary of the system. This is an oversimplification, as feedback can be contained within the system, or within smaller processes within the whole organization. For example, a measure of the effectiveness of measles immunization could be the local figures for deaths from measles, or the practice's figures for numbers of measles cases seen (outcome measures), or indirectly from the percentage of children in the practice immunized against measles (process measure). This corresponds to internal audit or performance review considered in Chapter 18.

Let us now look inside the boundary of the open system, and consider in more detail the processes which take place.

The main ingredients are:

1. *The tasks* and the technology to carry them out – what are we doing and how?

2. *The structure* in which work is done, which includes buildings, working structures such as teams, as well as the standards and procedures which govern the work.

3. *The people*, with their individual attitudes, values, skills, and relationships.

Although these three ingredients are part of the system, they are influenced by the environment, and in turn influence it. This is an interaction, not just a passive response. The point has been made elsewhere in the book that the practice tasks must relate to the demands and needs of the population served; but equally, patient demand can be influenced by education and other factors. The way a team works can be affected by the structure of the building and by restrictions or encouragement from nurse management. The people who work in an organization apply values from outside, and are all members of communities which may or may not impinge upon the practice.

Though the system has been subdivided into the three ingredients of task, structure, and people, these are mutually dependent, and any change in one affects the others.

A balanced approach to task, structure, and people will be more likely to succeed than, say, an emphasis on interpersonal relationships to the neglect of tasks, or vice versa.

There are, in addition, the linking processes which bring the whole organization to life, such as communicating, priority setting, resolving conflicts and

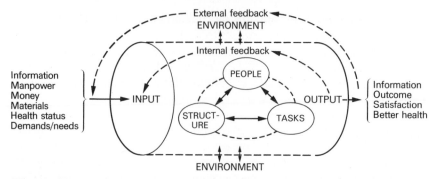

Fig. 16.6. The ingredients and processes of an open system. Arrows denote interaction, connecting lines and dashed lines denote linking processes, e.g. setting priorities, communication, collaboration, decision-making, problem-solving, and resolving conflicts.

solving problems (see Fig. 16.6). Some of these processes have been considered already, and others are considered in subsequent sections.

RESOLVING CONFLICTS

An organization entirely free of conflict would be a dull place to work, and could lead to boredom and a lack of creativity. Too much conflict can distort priorities, interfere with tasks, and make structures ineffective. How can we obtain the optimum level of conflict? This topic has been considered in the first three chapters, and the practice manager in her role as intermediary may be helped by considering the systems model, and its message to the inter-relationship of factors leading to conflict. It is easy to conclude that people have 'personality problems', when the cause of conflict lies in the task or structure domain, or the linking processes have broken down. If severe conflicts are unresolved, it is easy for warring camps to form, who see each other in unreal terms. The more they are made to co-operate, the more their misconceptions and stereotypes of one another are confirmed.

When conflicts occur it may be helpful for the manager to consider whether the needs of the people in conflict are being met satisfactorily. One way of looking at these needs is in terms of:

(1) identity;
(2) territory;
(3) control.

(Huntington 1981).

Each of us needs to be aware of our place in the organization, and to have a clear perception of our role and tasks. Territory is defended aggressively, and this term can cover the sole use of space, such as an office or a desk, as well as 'ownership' of tasks and patients. A measure of control of our own stake in the

organization is necessary for us all. Any imbalance of control between individuals or changes in the status quo may lead to conflict.

Many conflicts appear in one area, when the real origin is in another. An
experienced manager will determine the root cause of a conflict, and will try to
use it diagnostically and creatively to improve things as a whole; not just treat
the presenting symptom, or try to avoid conflict at all costs.

SOLVING PROBLEMS

However well we plan and manage, things do not always run smoothly. As
stated by the famous Murphy in his 3rd Law 'In any field of endeavour, anything that can go wrong, will go wrong'. One hopes that readers of this book
will not share Murphy's pressimism or bad luck, or is it really bad management?
Many of the chapters have dealt with solving problems in certain areas, but are
there any general guidelines which can help us?

As in medicine, prevention is better than cure, and the object of good
planning and management is to prevent problems arising by forestalling them,
or not letting the conditions arise in which problems are likely (e.g. by good
staff selection).

Some people, by their temperament, find it difficult to plan ahead, and
prefer to wait for trouble then deal with it with masterly decision. This is called
crisis management. Some people may thrive on it, but the organization is
bound to suffer. When unforeseen problems arise, then quick decisions are
needed. Because time is short, people do not usually gather together all the
information needed for a rational decision – they jump in with an answer. In
other words they treat before diagnosis. This is one of the commonest failings
of crisis management.

Doctors in their training are taught to diagnose before they treat. They spend
every consultation solving problems presented to them by their patients. In the
process they develop their own problem-solving model, an example of which is
described in the *Manual of primary health care* (Pritchard 1981). This model
has much in common with models developed for solving problems in industry.
On this reasoning, GPs should be very good at solving problems in the practice,
provided they can go through the process of collecting information in order to
decide what the problem is and its most likely cause, before putting forward a
tentative solution.

This step-by-step process does not suit everyone, but it is valuable to have
such a check-list in the background to ensure that nothing has been forgotten.
A practice manager needs this extra dimension of thoroughness in looking at a
problem from all sides, which gives her confidence in proposing and implementing a solution. Few problems are black and white, so greater discrimination is needed between the shades of grey.

The problem-solving model described here is an abbreviation of the one
developed for industry by Kepner and Tregoe, and described in their book *The*

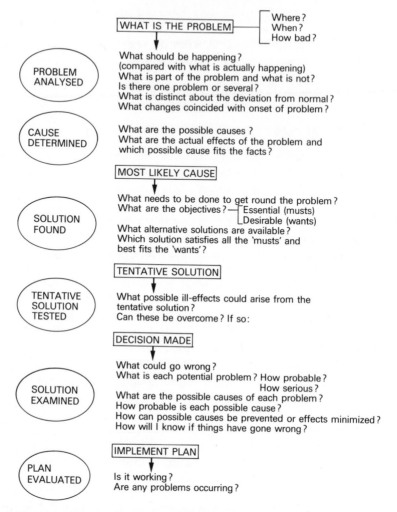

Fig. 16.7. Industrial problem-solving model. (Modified from Kepner and Tregoe (1981).)

new rational manager (Kepner and Tregoe 1981), which should be consulted in the original. This model (see Fig. 16.7) needs to be interpreted flexibly. It may be helpful for checking that no essential stages in solving a problem have been missed, resulting in a faulty diagnosis leading to the wrong treatment.

The early stages of analysing the problem are important, particularly in separating the real problem from the confusion of related problems, and pin-pointing the nature of the deviation from the expected, which is at the heart of the problem. Next comes the familiar question (to GPs) about what changes coincided with the onset of the problem. For example, did it always happen the minute the practice manager went on holiday?

Possible causes must be explored, the options weighed up, and the temptation to jump to conclusions resisted. The same applies to possible solutions. Sometimes people have a favourite solution, just waiting for a problem to turn up! A solution in search of a problem is a familiar pitfall for managers.

Once a solution has been selected, its likely side-effects must be examined, so that the treatment is not worse than the disease. Then the solution becomes a plan which needs to be implemented and evaluated. These are the topics of the next two chapters.

Insoluble problems

Some problems seem so difficult from the start that the people involved shy away from them. An alternative is to seek outside help. A GP or practice manager who has had a similar problem might join in a discussion from which progress could be made. Or an expert might be called in. He or she might be a management consultant experienced in the field of primary health care, or a management services officer, or an operational research specialist. It is likely that the RHA or DHA would know of a management consultant whose fee could be afforded (ca: £400 a day). Alternatively, the RHA may employ an organization development consultant who might be seconded to the practice for a certain number of sessions. He or she would probably join in practice meetings to discuss the problem, and would act in a facilitative role, rather than impose or suggest an expert solution which might not be acceptable. The facilitator would help the mutual learning process which is the basis of planning and problem-solving. Most Regional, and some District Health Authorities have management services and operational research units which might help with more technical management problems. They, too, work with the people on the spot towards an agreed solution.

The general term for this activity is 'Action Research', in which the process of enquiry produces subtle changes which may illuminate the problem and lead the way to a solution. One method is for the researcher to interview all the people involved in a problem, and collect their views and ideas together. These are then fed back to the group in a summary, without disclosing people's names. The resulting discussion may lead to new insights into the problem and consequent action.

All the methods described are aimed at improving the problem-solving skills of the people doing the job, not to make them dependent on experts.

If practices have run out of problems, they might try making plans to solve, or forestall, disasters such as the building being destroyed by fire, or the medical records being stolen! Then if it happened, the shock would be less severe.

17 Making plans

Much of this book has been about thinking ahead, seeing the wider picture, and reviewing our progress – about being in charge, rather than being overtaken by events. In Chapter 7, looking to the future and managing change was considered. In this chapter we take a more formal look at planning, and try to draw on the experience of people who have had to plan in other fields, both inside and outside the NHS. As well as looking at planning at the practice level, we must not forget that we are on the receiving end of plans made (or not made) at district, regional, and national levels.† Is there anything we can do to ensure that these, more central, plans meet our aspirations?

Later parts of this chapter may be of less concern to practice managers, but are more relevant to those GPs who involve themselves in NHS management in management teams or as authority members.

Why plan at all?

General practice and primary health care are complex areas of great uncertainty, in which prediction and planning are difficult. Why should we bother to plan? Why not wait for events to make action urgent, so that we have to move, by which time the answer may be clearer? This is a transparent fallacy, in which an analogy from medicine might help. Do we wait for a patient with abdominal pain to develop an acute abdomen before we act? Is there no chance that early diagnosis will make the patient's survival more likely and the treatment less painful? By acting early do we not keep our options open, giving ourselves room for manoeuvre and choice? By waiting for the crisis, we have no choice.

So let us try to plan, but accept that we cannot plan for all eventualities, and that some crises will occur. When they do, we will be more ready for them, and will have some problem-solving ideas and methods worked out.

What model of primary health care is appropriate?

It is helpful to start with some idea how primary health care (PHC) functions, so that we can study its working, and make predictions of its future behaviour. Does it work like a small business, or a machine, or a football team, or a local government department? We would probably all agree that primary health care is a complex biological system, involving many people with different roles and aims, working in a changing society with all its pressures and interactions. The

†The examples of NHS planning are taken in the context of England. The principles apply equally in the other countries of the United Kingdom.

most appropriate way to look at this type of arrangement is probably to regard it as an *open system*, as described in Chapter 16 (see Fig. 16.6).

How can we use the model to help us plan our work? It helps us to see the parts which make up the whole, and to study each in turn to ensure that our planning is comprehensive – a sort of check-list. We are reminded of the constituents of team working, and of the processes involved, all of which play their part in an effective system. The model draws our attention to the need for measures of input and outcome, and feedback of information for planning. Information is also needed about the social milieu in which the practice works, and about the technology it uses.

In previous chapters we have emphasized the complexity of the interactions between the people, the tasks, and the structure in which they work, as well as the many and varied processes of interaction. To summarize this in a simple diagram does not make the difficulties disappear, but gives a foundation on which to build our knowledge and experience – a unifying concept which gives us confidence in an uncertain world. Whilst not providing an easy answer to our problems, it can be used as a frame of reference for the mutual learning process which planning involves. By testing our ideas against the model, we challenge both our ideas and the model. If there is a mismatch we can modify our ideas or modify the model, or both.

PLANNING AT PRACTICE LEVEL

In Chapter 7 the difficulties of coping with change were described, and ways of looking into the future and managing change were discussed, as well as practice objectives and policies. All these are the groundwork of planning. To take it a stage further we must ask:

(1) where are we now? (and it may be helpful to ask how we arrived here);
(2) where do we want to go, and why?
(3) how do we get there?
(4) how do we know if or when we have got there?
(5) what next?

Where are we now? (and how did we arrive here?)

Firstly, we can look at the open system model (Fig. 16.6 and Table 7.1) and see if we can answer questions such as these:

1. What information do we have about our present position? Is it enough? What further information do we need? Can we get it?

2. What is the present position in terms of manpower, of revenue, capital, buildings, equipment, demand, and need for health care?

3. Do we have enough information about the situation in the environment (e.g. changes in population, age structure, ethnic mix, expectations, etc?)

4. What tasks are we undertaking now, and are the structure, people, and processes adequate for the tasks?

5. What information do we have about the results of our efforts? Is this information fed back and used?

6. How did we get here? History sometimes helps us to gauge the resistance to change which we are likely to meet.

Where do we want to go?

1. Why do we want to go there?

2. What are our overall goals and why are they our goals?

3. What more detailed and limited objectives do we have, and over what sort of time scale?

4. What are the relative priorities of our objectives?

The time scale is important. Planning for ten years ahead is valuable, but can be in broad terms only, covering *general strategy*; it is unlikely that enough information will be available for detailed planning. The shorter-term planning can be called tactical or *operational planning*. Table 7.1 gives a framework for strategic planning. In this section we will concentrate on the more immediate operational planning, such as screening or immunization programmes (see Appendices A–D).

How do we get there?

This sounds more like the planning considered in previous chapters. Having set our objectives, priorities, and time scale, what are the next steps? Traditional management teaching suggests that there are four main elements:

(1) make a plan;

(2) motivate the people involved;

(3) put the plan into action;

(4) evaluate its success and re-plan.

Each element has several steps, as shown in Table 17.1. This check-list does not cover every situation, but it will act as a reminder to those making the plan, so that essential steps are not forgotten – such as discussing the plan with the people who have to carry it out! Responsibilities must be clearly spelled out, and written procedures developed. Unless people understand their place in the scheme, they will be confused and not give of their best.

Planning needs to be a joint exercise involving everybody who has something to contribute to its implementation. All must be persuaded of the value of the plan to the practice and patients as a whole, and to each of them individually. 'What's in it for me?' is a valid question, though the benefit to the individual may be an indirect one, such as sharing in the aims of a well-motivated working group.

A simpler model of planning is shown in Fig. 17.1. It requires the people involved to describe their present situation, and their desired goal for the future, and plan how to get there. The next step is to identify all the circum-

Table 17.1. *Operational planning check-list*

A. *Steps in formulating plan*
   1. What are the objectives we want to achieve and why?
   2. What background information have we about the situation, and can it be relied upon?
   3. *How* can objectives be met?
       Are there alternative solutions?
       What methods have others tried – have they been effective?
       Can their plans be modified to suit present situation?
   4. What are the consequences of the different options?
   5. What differences in cost – manpower
                           – cash
                           – other resources
   6. Weigh up options and list in order of preference.
   7. Decide on preferred plan.

B. *Steps in motivating*
   1. Provide background knowledge to give point to the plan.
   2. Where appropriate involve all staff in formulating plan and deciding on options (minimally A6 and 7).
   3. Present preferred plan to all staff and invite comments and suggestions. Discuss with patients' representatives if possible.
   4. Modify plan in the light of staff and patients' suggestions.
   5. Discuss any training or equipment needed.

C. *Steps in carrying out plan*
   1. Devise detailed procedures if possible in form of algorithm (or decision tree) to cover all possibilities, in consultation with staff concerned.
   2. Fix starting date, decide rate of progress, completion date and any subsequent action.
   3. Identify and allocate responsibilities (i.e. 'who does what'). Train staff where necessary.
   4. Order equipment.

D. *Steps in evaluation*
   1. Fix times to evaluate.
   2. Have objectives been achieved? If not, to what extent has there been shortfall in quantity, quality, or time? Has experience suggested modification?
   3. Has plan been found faulty and have modifications been made? Have these been effective?
   4. Have other objectives been generated from experience gained in carrying out and evaluating plan?

From Pritchard, P. (1981) *Manual of primary health care.* 2nd Edn. Oxford University Press, Oxford.

stances and people who may help them reach their goal, and all the circumstances and people hindering progress. Having defined the helping and hindering forces, they can plan to gain from the former and circumvent the latter. This method sometimes goes by the jargon name of 'force field analysis', but readers should not let the name deter them from trying a useful method of studying the factors influencing change.

For those who like setting out their data in graphic form, the factors may be written in, and the strength of their influence on progress indicated by the length or thickness of the arrow.

Implementing plans means doing things differently, and implies a change of behaviour. It is a learning process in which we all have to participate, in order to ensure success.

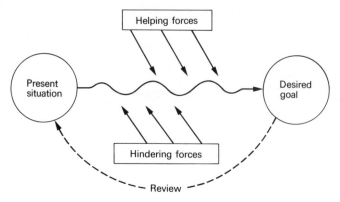

Fig. 17.1. A planning model.

How do we know if or when we have got there, and what next?

How often is this essential element omitted or glossed over? The subject of feedback or taking stock is stressed in Chapter 18. It is of particular importance where there is a formal plan with a time scale, which then probably leads on to other plans. These new aims may well arise when experience of carrying out the plan changes our thinking. Alternatively, the plan might have been one in a list of priorities, and we need to choose when to divert our energy to the next priority on the list. Some of these points have been covered in the check list (Table 17.1).

So far we have discussed planning at practice level, regarding the practice as a fairly autonomous unit which can decide its own destiny. Many plans need the co-operation of attached staff such as nurses, whose managers need to be involved and to agree to the proposed changes. Some plans may involve more than one practice, and so be appropriate to the level of the District Community Unit. We now consider the next planning level.

PLANNING AT DISTRICT LEVEL

Primary health care services are partly administered by the District Health Authority, and partly by the Family Practitioner Committee. Whereas the 1974 NHS re-organization attempted some integration of these two bodies, the 1982 re-organization has tended to isolate them from each other.

Social Services, which were planned to work closely with Area Health Authorities through joint consultative committees, and with general practice through attachment schemes, have tended to become more remote. As well as the organizational obstacles, they are suffering severe financial cuts.

The District Health Authority (DHA)

This authority serves a population of quarter to half a million people. Their policy is decided by their members (mostly lay, but including a GP, a nurse and a consultant) on the advice of their team of officers, (District Administrator, District Treasurer, District Medical Officer, and District Nursing Officer) and led by the District General Manager (DGM).

Some districts delegate administration to units, such as a large hospital. In most cases the community services are administered as a separate unit. These units also have general managers.

DHA community services

The major DHA community services are listed below:

Health visiting
District nursing
District midwifery
Physiotherapy
Chiropody
Child health clinics and other services for children
School medical service
Services for physically and mentally handicapped
Family planning clinics
Medical support for social services
Health education
Works services and supplies
Community hospitals (including GP maternity units)
Health centre building (delegated from RHA)
Health centre staffing and maintenance
Specialized nursing services in the community (often hospital-based) e.g. psychiatric, paediatric, geriatric, diabetic, stoma-care, etc.
Supervision of nursing homes
Staff education and training

The DHA has to budget strictly for all their services. Different budgets cover medical staff, nursing staff, administrative staff, maintenance of buildings, and the specialist nursing based on hospitals. It is difficult to plan effectively when services are not integrated.

Community health councils (CHCs) operate at district level, and have to be consulted by DHAs before implementing their plans. This is the most effective level at which the patient's voice can be heard, and plans negotiated. For all their lack of resources and planning experience, some CHCs are making a very useful impact, though their progress is slow in some districts. CHCs are an unique experiment, and are attracting considerable interest worldwide.

The Family Practitioner Committee (FPC)

The FPC is independent of the DHA. It is accountable to the Secretary of State. In the past the chairman and vice chairman were elected by the members; in future, both are likely to be appointed by the Secretary of State. Members have, in the past, been appointed by Area Health Authorities (now defunct), professional advisory bodies, and local authorities. The future pattern of membership is unclear at the time of writing. FPCs receive their budget from the DHSS, and much of it is 'open ended'.

FPCs are responsible for the family practitioner services, including:

(1) general medical practitioners;
(2) general dental practitioners;
(3) ophthalmic medical practitioners and ophthalmic opticians;
(4) dispensing chemists.

In the area of general medical practitioner services they administer all the services described in the 'Red Book', and the GPs' terms of service. The FPC is advised by a Local Medical Committee (LMC) in relation to general medical services. The LMC nominates (at present) eight members of the FPC. There are in addition seven other professional members and 15 lay members (11 appointed by the health authority, and four by local authority). The structure and functions of FPCs are set out in more detail in the booklet by Parr and Williams (1981).†

Local Authority Services

Personal Social Services are provided by the Social Services Department of the local authority. These include:

(1) social workers in area teams, general practice and hospitals;
(2) home helps, friendly neighbours, etc.;
(3) meals on wheels;
(4) services for the disabled e.g. home alterations, appliances, occupational therapy;
(5) day centres and luncheon clubs for elderly.

In addition, social services provide residential care for the elderly, physically and mentally handicapped, and children in need of care.

The importance of co-ordinating these services with medical services was a cornerstone of the 1974 re-organization and to make this easier their boundaries were the same wherever possible. With the abolition of the area tier in 1982 and the blurring of district boundaries, co-operation was made more difficult. To achieve co-ordination of services at practice and district level

†*Family Practitioner Services and their administration* (1981). Parr, C. W. and Williams, J. P. Institute of Health Service Managers, 75 Portland Place, London, W1N 4AN.

requires much greater effort, and closer than ever links between general practice and social work.

District Councils usually provide housing, including sheltered housing and the appointment of Wardens.

Working together

Integrated planning of the care of (for example) the elderly may now involve the following people and authorities:

(1) General Practitioner;
(2) Health Visitor;
(3) District Nurse, and nursing aide;
(4) other members of the primary health-care team;
(5) social worker (in PHC or area team);
(6) home helps and other personal social services;
(7) geriatric liaison health visitor;
(8) District Council sheltered housing;
(9) social services residential or day care;
(10) Community hospital services;
(11) geriatric hospital services – inpatient, outpatient, or day ward;
(12) psychiatric hospital and community services;
(13) voluntary agencies and private residential homes;
(14) Community Health Council.

The various authorities may be pursuing different policies, and integrated planning is the exception rather than the rule. All have their separate budgets which are subject to cash limits, with the exception of the FPC. The boundaries of care (i.e. whether an old person should be in her home, sheltered housing, local authority, or hospital residential care) are so imprecise that there is a tendency for each authority to hope that someone else will provide care. The result is underprovision, and the build-up of need for care in the community. The primary health-care team and facilities have to cope with the extra load, so it is in all their interests to understand clearly how the system works, whose responsibility it is to do what, and ways of bringing pressure to bear on the various services to provide appropriate care. The burden of care falls chiefly on families, but they have little input into planning, except through the agency of the CHC, or national pressure groups.

District planning for prevention

In spite of all the difficulties inherent in the structure of health and social services, some districts have developed close liaison, and integrated plans for certain care groups, such as the elderly, mentally ill, mentally handicapped, physically handicapped, and children. To orient these planning teams in the direction of prevention is far-sighted, but all the more difficult with over-loaded 'caring and curing' services.

General practitioners do not find it easy to conform to a district plan, unless they see some benefit to themselves and their patients. The plan must be shown to benefit their practice, and must be presented to the general practitioners in an acceptable form, preferably by one of their number. Some authorities have recruited 'GP-facilitators' to try to co-ordinate the work of several practices in implementing a particular programme. Examples of such programmes are:

1. To help general practitioners with the formidable administrative work involved in improving their premises.

2. To help GPs and the PHC team to develop preventive programmes in their practices (e.g. arterial disease, smoking, hypertension, cervical cytology, immunization).

3. To help in the development of practice computerization as an aid to the preventive programmes.

4. To support health-education projects based on the PHC team.

5. To use educational methods to develop more effective team working.

6. To encourage general practitioners to develop shared care (e.g. diabetics and hypertensives).

7. To help and support general practitioners in auditing their prescribing.

The emphasis is on support for initiatives in primary health care which suit the particular practice circumstances, not a standardized 'take it or leave it' scheme. General practitioners who will be helping to implement a plan must be encouraged to contribute ideas at an early stage, and be involved in its development.

DHAs have a duty to ascertain the health status of the population served, as well as the levels and effectiveness of care. Up to now these measures have been applied erratically, and have not involved close liaison with PHC. Equally, any programmes based on primary health care, such as those listed above, will need to be evaluated and the results fed back to the PHC teams. Unless health-care practice is measured against the health of the population served, we may delude ourselves into thinking we are doing good just because we are busy. That is to say, we are measuring an unevaluated process rather than an objective outcome.

Planning at area or district level has tended to concentrate on 'norms' of provision based on national averages, or what was considered desirable. This was expressed in numbers of beds per 1000 population in the various specialties, and numbers of nurses and other staff. There were no measures of efficiency, or of the effectiveness of the care given in terms of curing disease or improving health. People believed that what they were doing was right, so the policy was to spread it evenly or do more of it.

In the past ten years an attempt has been made to relate the planning process more to 'care groups' such as the elderly, the mentally handicapped, the mentally ill, children, accident and emergency, and general surgery, and try to measure the efficiency of use of resources in terms of cases treated per bed, and cost per case. Unless the use of resources is related to outcome, we are no further along the road to rational planning.

Primary health care figured little in the plans (except in numbers of health centres and community nurses) because there were no good measures of effectiveness and efficiency, little financial control, and (in the case of the independent contractors) no managerial control. In spite of these structural barriers to planning, some progress has been made in integrating hospital and primary health care. To achieve this integration there must be co-operation between the FPC, the Local Medical Committee, the local faculty of the RCGP, the post-graduate dean and tutors, and at District Headquarters the District Management Team, the Planning Officer, the Community Nursing Officer, and the Community Medical Officers.

Commitment to integrated planning of PHC must be more than just words. Such an initiative costs money to get it started (pump-priming). It would be hoped that the implementation of preventive policies would save much more than the initial cost, but this would take time.

PLANNING AT REGIONAL LEVEL

The 14 regions in England† receive the district plans and co-ordinate them in relation to the resources likely to be available for the region, in relation to regional policies, and in response to national guidelines. Following negotiation, and modification where needed, plans are approved and resources are allocated to districts.

Major capital schemes are planned at the Regional Health Authority (RHA), and these form a part of the ten-year regional strategic plan. In spite of firm statements about the need to develop primary health care, from Secretaries of State downwards, the level of resources devoted to it has fallen in relation to expenditure in other parts of the health services.‡ Many regions would like to see PHC expenditure increased, but find it hard to argue a case for its cost-effectiveness in the face of pressing demands for new coronary-care and accident units, or more pacemakers. PHC plans must fit in with national priorities which favour the elderly, the mentally ill, and mentally handicapped (see *care in action*, a handbook of policies and priorities for health and personal social services in England. DHSS 1981).

It is rare for the regional plans to show any integrated statistics for PHC, that is combining the FPC figures with those of other community services such as district nursing and health visiting.

† Different arrangements apply in Scotland, Wales, and Northern Ireland.

‡ For example, general medical services in 1986 received just over 7 per cent of the total NHS revenue, whereas in 1970 it was over 8 per cent, and in 1954 it was 10 per cent. The actual revenue has increased over the years (at constant prices), but the hospital costs have risen at a much higher rate. (see Office of Health Economics *Compendium of health statistics*, 6th edn., 1987). There has, however, been some increase in the numbers of health visitors and district nurses.

There has been a change in the usage of hospital beds over the past ten years, with a much shorter hospital stay for patients, and generally more intensive use of hospital facilities. Earlier discharge of hospital patients and more care in the community (e.g. psychiatric patients and the elderly) has put greater demands on the community nursing services and general practice, which has not been met by a comparable increase in resources. Whether standards of care in the community have fallen as a result is hard to judge, in the absence of clear indicators of quality.

The challenge to planners at regional level is considerable. They can meet it only if practical plans for development of primary health care and improving health are initiated in individual practices, co-ordinated and supported at district level, and sent on to region for incorporation in the regional plan.

Though emphasis has been placed in this chapter on the needs of PHC, it should not be forgotten that it can only function as part of an integrated and co-ordinated district and national service.

PLANNING AT NATIONAL LEVEL

The further one travels from the individual patient and the individual practice, the harder it becomes to make plans which are practical and meet local needs. Thus the challenge to planners at national level is even greater. What are the specific requirements of national planning for primary health care? The World Health Organization suggests the following:

(1) a national policy for health;
(2) a national priority for developing primary health care;
(3) intersectoral collaboration at all levels;
(4) community involvement at all levels;
(5) development of programmes where these are appropriate to national planning (e.g. immunization, cervical screening, child health, maternity);
(6) decentralization of planning and management of services as far as possible;
(7) development of management support for primary health care.

National policy for health

Good health is not just a product of good medical care, but is more dependent on economic development, employment levels, wages, housing, good environmental conditions, and a healthy individual lifestyle. Unless a co-ordinated plan for health embraces all these factors, success in achieving optimum health of the population is unlikely.

An example of confusion about a national policy for health is the absence of a co-ordinated policy for dealing with today's major threat to health – smoking. The Treasury gains from taxation, and shorter life expectancy of its smoking pensioners; the Department of Industry subsidizes the building of tobacco factories; the Ministry of Sport allows tobacco sponsorship of sporting events to have wide media coverage; and a powerful tobacco-industry lobby in Parliament is allowed to delay legislation. All the time the Department of Health does its best under these difficult circumstances. Unless a health policy is agreed at cabinet level, the opportunities for inter-departmental procrastination are infinite, and no policy results. The Health Education Council tries to compete with tobacco industry promotion on a much smaller budget.

National priority for developing primary health care

The World Health Organization (WHO/UNICEF 1978) is strongly committed to developing primary health care as the most effective and economical way of improving a nation's health. They specify that primary health care must include health promotion and prevention of illness as priorities over the provision of acceptable and affordable accessible health care. The member states of WHO (including the United Kingdom) have endorsed this policy, but not yet implemented it. It is more difficult to implement where there is a strongly entrenched, efficient, and popular *medical* (rather than *health*) care system which takes first priority for resources. Professional entrenchment is strongest in medical-student education which is completely specialist-dominated, except in a few forward-looking medical schools. The NHS, as it functions at present, would be more appropriately named a national sickness service. Within its limitations it gives good value for money, but is it the best way to spend the money if the primary objective is improving the nation's health?

Intersectoral collaboration at all levels

Mention has been made of the need for a national policy involving all the agencies which are relevant to health, (e.g. employment, housing, social work). For this to be effective, there must be collaboration between them at national, regional, district, and practice levels. Such collaboration is unlikely to take place unless the structural arrangements are laid down by statute, and are backed up by the political will to ensure co-operation and co-ordination. Particularly strong policies are needed to ensure that 'under-served groups' like the mentally handicapped, receive their share of resources. However, while waiting for the creation of statutory powers, informal collaboration can be encouraged.

Community involvement at all levels

Community participation takes many forms and operates at many levels. Whether this participation is real or just a token is open to question. Patients tend to accept what services are provided, which encourages apathy, whereas participation and involvement in providing a service is more likely to result in an active interest in ways of achieving good health. The success and growth of self-help and disability or disease groups is a measure of the extent, energy, and resources which the community is prepared to contribute.

At practice level, patient participation groups perform a similar function to

CHCs at district level, but only about one practice in 100 has such a group. In spite of minimal official support, the number of patient groups in general practice is expanding rapidly.

Regional health authorities tend to liaise with CHCs, but there are no statutory links at this level. At DHSS level there is no formal patient involvement in planning, though some advisory committees have appointed lay members. Another unique British institution is 'Question Time' in the House of Commons, when Ministers responsible may be questioned by Members of Parliament. Though a valuable bastion of freedom and a safety valve, it may distort priorities and is not the same as community participation in planning.

Development of national programmes

Uniformity of service is desirable wherever one happens to live, and certain national PHC programmes have been developed, though operational implementation is a local responsibility. Examples are child immunization, cervical screening, family planning, and maternity services. Where services are carried out by general practitioners an 'item of service' fee may be paid. Naturally the DHSS is reluctant to add any new fees to the list, so changes are slow, and desirable policies – such as general practitioners doing more health promotion or minor surgery – are not encouraged.

Decentralization of planning and management of services

It is generally agreed that locally planned and managed services can be more efficient and more responsive to need, though their quality may vary from district to district. The DHSS has to balance the need for central accountability against the stifling of local initiative. The policy is to delegate planning and management to districts as far as possible, but to maintain some monitoring system to ensure that acceptable standards are maintained. This has not proved an easy task, as suitable indicators of quality are few and far between. Some progress has been made in applying transatlantic accreditation techniques to individual hospital units and districts in England. But no uniform system of ensuring the quality of primary health-care services has yet been developed, though voluntary peer-audit (or performance review) is gaining ground.

It is up to practices and districts to put their house in order and aim at high standards, rather than have arbitrary and rigid standards imposed from the centre. A public service cannot escape public accountability.

The NHS Planning System

The NHS planning system is based on a long-term (10–15 year) strategic view of objectives, priorities, and resources, with a three-yearly revision of plans. Operational planning works on a one-year cycle.

The DHSS produces guidelines for national policy, based on expert advice, political considerations, and likely availability of resources. In response to these guidelines, modified where necessary by RHAs, the DHAs make their plans which then go back up the ladder. This is shown in diagrammatic form in Fig. 17.2. The recent (1982) re-organization of the NHS, abolished the Area Health Authority tier, and added a district general manager (DGM).

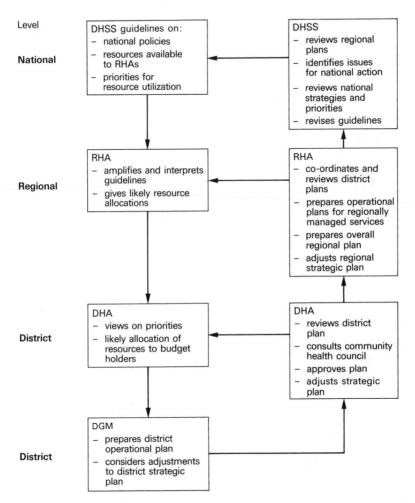

Fig. 17.2. The NHS planning cycle. (Modified from OHE, 1977). *The reorganized NHS.* Office of Health Economics, 12 Whitehall, London SW1A 2DY.)

These changes have re-opened the question of the effectiveness of the national planning system. Is a centralized planning system bound to be in-efficient and insensitive to local needs? Bureaucracy is an essential feature of centralized planning, but can it be made effective, flexible, innovative, and humane? Or does it inevitably lead to a risk-avoidance exercise, which discourages innovation, and leads to organizational stagnation? The record of the NHS in terms of innovation (new and different) has not been as good as its ability to maintain and improve existing services (more and better). †

Development of management support for primary health care

The lack of a planning function for FPCs has been mentioned, and it is typical of the relative lack of management support for general practice compared with hospital or health authority services. This picture is now changing, and the DHSS is giving considerable support to management-training courses for general practitioners and employed staff. For integrated management support for primary health care at district and regional level, further initiatives will be needed. The unit management concept introduced at the 1982 re-organization should include a community sector or unit serving GPs, attached and employed staff, and community hospitals. For this purpose administrators skilled in this field will be needed, as well as other supporting staff.

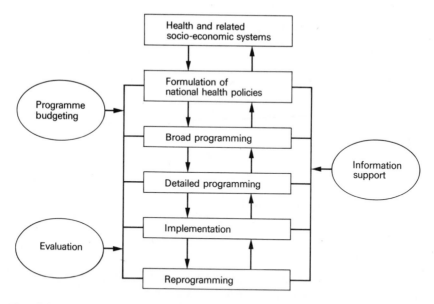

Fig. 17.3. Managerial process for national health development. (From World Health Organization (1981). *Managerial process for national health development.* Health for All Series No. 5. WHO, Geneva.)

---

† From a paper presented by a working group of the Royal Institute of Public Administration at a conference at the King's Fund Centre, 28 October 1981. King's Fund Report KFC 82/7.

THE WORLD HEALTH ORGANIZATION VIEWPOINT

The World Health Organization, in its programme of 'Health for all by the year 2000', has made several detailed studies of the development of national programmes for improving health. Though their emphasis has been on developing countries, the general concepts have been confirmed for industrialized countries. The guiding principles for the success of these programmes, outlined already, are not considered in detail here. The WHO model however, has so much in common with the planning steps described earlier in this chapter, that it is shown as Fig. 17.3. Its chief difference from the NHS planning model is the broadly-based top policy level, involving health and related socio-economic systems.

The increasing tempo of World Health Organization impact on primary health care, the 1982 NHS re-organization, severe cash shortages, demographic changes, and the major changes taking place in general practice itself will all ensure that the next ten years will be as challenging to planners, as to service providers. Can we afford to let things drift, or must we accept the challenge in order to provide maximum improvement in peoples' health, and optimum provision of health care to meet need as well as demand? Above all, how can we ensure an acceptable quality of life for those who are ill?

18 Reviewing performance

WHAT IS REVIEW?

The term 'review' is borrowed from the world of business, where output per man and profits can be measured and reviewed from time to time. The health field is much more complex, with less tangible indicators of performance. But without a review of performance, as mentioned in Chapter 17, the organization cannot hold its course towards its objective.

As described in Chapter 16, businesses tend to adopt a hierarchical organization with the boss at the top of the pyramid, and a chain of authority spreading from him to the periphery. General practitioners are independent of any direct chain of command, and work in a team context with nursing staff who are themselves subject to higher authority. The general practitioner in his turn is the boss as far as his direct employees are concerned. The result is a very complex organization, in which the only feasible method of review is a voluntary one of self-audit, or peer-review in small groups such as the partners, or the team. Review, as shown in Fig. 17.1, relates output to input, both of the whole organization, and of the sub-units of which it is made up. Each sub-unit can be seen as a 'mini-system' with its own input, process, and output, and contributing to the total organization. To review the total system in terms of benefit to the health of patients is difficult. We may have to content ourselves with sub-divisions of the total output (e.g. immunization rate or patient-satisfaction), or with the efficiency of the process (e.g. the delay in the appointment system). The subjects under review fall broadly into two categories – organizational and clinical. The two categories overlap, in that good organization benefits the clinical care of patients, but in the small compass of this book, the emphasis is on audit (or review) of the organization rather than on clinical audit.

Whose responsibility

Because general practitioners are independent professionals, and are not subject to any systematic process of audit (with the exception of prescription costs, certification, and complaints), the onus is firmly on them to maintain standards. Nurses in primary health care also enjoy a higher level of autonomy than their colleagues in hospital, and have a responsibility for monitoring their own standards, but many of the tasks in general practice are undertaken jointly in a team setting, so a joint review is neeeded of the performance of these tasks.

How to do it

Tasks undertaken by an individual are amenable to self-review, but incentives are increased, and the critical edge is sharpened when review is carried out in small groups. How do we set about it? We have already described the need to define policies; to set objectives; to agree on standards that can be measured (performance indicators); to apply the criteria; to note any shortfall in achievement; and to take corrective action.

Without a clear aim, we just drift with the current. We may look around from time to time to see where we have drifted, which is perhaps better than drifting with firmly closed eyes, but such activity lacks purpose and control.

PERFORMANCE INDICATORS

Each objective will need to be described in terms of the level of achievement or behaviour by certain people in a given time. These may be described as targets, meaning a precisely defined objective to be achieved in a given time.

In the clinical field the aim might be to keep a patient's blood pressure below a certain level, and to check it at stated intervals. In the practice-management field we may not have such clear indicators of performance, but if we are to review performance at all, then we must look for best available indicators.

Without clear measures, we have the choice of just reviewing those areas of performance which are clearly measurable, or alternatively, trying to develop indicators to suit our needs. Much data can be collected in a practice, and often it is enough to do a spot check, rather than keep detailed and continuing statistics. For example, examine 30 medical records at random to see how many have missing dates of birth, incorrect addresses, or no record of blood pressure. Some measures, like staff morale and patient satisfaction have no easy yardsticks, but a subjective impression is better than nothing. Such measures are known as 'qualitative' and imply a value judgement, such as the quality of care. They do not have the same respectability as the numerical or 'quantitative' measures of which statistics are made. But which is more important to a patient – the quality of life (or care) or the numerical level of a statistic? This lack of agreed indicators presents a serious dilemma for general practice. Do we just measure such things as immunization rates, or try to do a bit of soul-searching about the quality of care? If we only collect hard and measurable data, we may miss the things which really matter.

An eminent health statistician has stated that if you select the highest possible quality of staff, give them the best possible training, and keep their morale high – the quality of health care will look after itself. This statement stresses the importance of the people giving care rather than 'numbers of patients treated', with no measure of how well or thoroughly they were treated.

Internal or external audit

The trend in North America is to develop highly sophisticated methods for measuring health care, with teams of experienced observers putting hospitals and family medicine services under the microscope in order that they may be 'accredited'. This is a valuable example of external audit, as distinct from individual or small-group review (internal audit). However, the imminence of an external audit, concentrates people's minds on internal audit or self-review, but one element is usually missing from external audit and that is a consumer view. Recipients of health care, or members of a community may not be able to produce many statistics, but they have a viewpoint which is doubly valuable. First, their satisfaction is what health care is all about, and secondly, their views may add a new and important dimension to a purely professional evaluation. The World Health Organization has sponsored many projects for 'community evaluation'; patients sit on the General Medical Council, and on local ethical committees; and patient participation is spreading (as described in Chapter 6).

PUTTING PERFORMANCE REVIEW TO WORK

Having developed indicators of a particular performance, they must be applied in an agreed manner at an agreed time. Shortfall in achievement must be recorded, and the people concerned informed about it. The next stage is to discuss what to do, and so set off another cycle of planning to new objectives, new achievements, and new policies. It is a continuing process, with a strong educational content. Just to measure performance has a subtle effect on that performance, known as the 'halo' or Hawthorne effect, which may upset researchers but is likely to please the consumer.

THE PRACTICE MANAGER'S ROLE IN PERFORMANCE REVIEW

Where does the practice manager start? First she can check through and list objectives, policies, and decisions, and rank them for priority, both in terms of their importance and their urgency. From this list a review schedule can be made. For each topic for review there must be performance indicators, target dates, etc., as described above. If it is something which the manager can review herself, she can get on with it, and record the result. Next she can inform the people concerned as to whether the review is favourable or unfavourable. In either case, it is a spur to do better. When the review is outside the manager's capability, then she must remind and coax the people who can do it. Equally, if she finds that objectives and priorities have not been decided upon, she must bring this to the partners' notice, and try to involve any other people who may be concerned in the review.

If the target has not been reached, new plans or a new time scale must be set, and a date for further review entered in the diary. Similarly, when targets are reached, the manager must help to formulate new objectives, targets, and plans. It is a never-ending process in general practice, because the work is never done. This open-ended commitment to care and the uncertainty of measures of achievement makes review all the more important, so that effort is conserved, priorities are set, and morale is maintained.

It is tempting to respond to crises and to do tasks as they arise, and then to find that there is no time left to do the really important checking as to whether all the effort has been effective.

Just as money must be found to invest in new equipment or buildings, so time must be found to invest in review as a step to improved effectiveness. Without the time, the practice manager will not be able to use her imagination to monitor the less obvious aspects of the work of the practice. She needs to do some 'lateral thinking' to explore the need for care, not just the demand; e.g. to find out how many people try to telephone the surgery and fail to get through, rather than just log telephone messages. Review and research are different words for the same process of enquiry – of learning from observation and experience, as a basis for informed action.

Monitoring performance implies the collection of data, and this is very much in the domain of the practice manager, whether it be statistics concerning finance or workload, or logs of appointments requested; these topics have been considered in previous chapters. Written records of policies, decisions, and rules have been mentioned, as has the diary as an aid to self discipline. The practice manager must decide how she ensures that the system really works – that the diary is checked, and omissions carried forward, and that decisions are carried out or brought back for further discussion.

Assessing the quality of leadership

When reviewing performance, the practice manager must show leadership by initiating review. One way is to examine the various systems and subsystems, as described earlier. Another is to examine whether people's needs in terms of identity, territory, and control are being met (see Chapter 16).

A different way of looking at leadership has been formulated by Vaill (1982) who describes the essentials of leadership in terms of:

(1) time;
(2) feeling;
(3) focus.

Time

Successful leaders work hard, but above all they use their time efficiently, and *find time* in a busy day, in order to do things which matter. This implies an order of priorities, which is part of 'focus'. As well as the tactical, short-term use of time, successful leaders think further ahead. They often stay longer in the same job, which helps them to take a longer view.

Feeling

This term reflects the way that good leaders really care about the way the organization runs, the service it gives, and the contentment of staff within it.

This feeling is a reflection of their values and philosophy, which good leaders will not keep to themselves. Though colleagues and subordinates may not share their intense commitment, some sense of common purpose must pervade the whole organization.

Focus

A clear sense of direction and of priorities is essential to leadership. The leader must focus on what she thinks the organization needs most — not necessarily the jobs which are most pleasant. This sense of priorities must be communicated to others in the organization as appropriate.

The qualities described might seem an ideal beyond the reach of ordinary mortals. But the concept is important in terms of the *balance* needed between the three factors, rather than the level of excellence in each. Indeed, too high a level of one factor unbalances the whole system. For example the general practitioner who works round the clock, and feels deeply for his or her work may well lack focus, so that leadership fails. The 'workaholic' may spend time in order to compensate for lack of feeling and focus. Some leaders may try to remain detached, in order to maintain their commitment of time and their sharp focus. They may be efficient, but this pattern is not found among successful leaders. Similarly, other imbalances of the three factors do not result in successful leadership, and a deficiency of all three factors is another way of describing the 'laissez-faire' leadership style described in Chapter 7.

As well as being systematic and conscientious in her checking, the practice manager must use her communication skills to ensure that she obtains the information she needs, and is keeping everyone in the organization informed about progress towards targets, and achievements — as well as shortcomings. In this way everyone in the organization shares responsibility for the overall outcome, and so develops a sense of pride based on reality rather than fantasy.

The practice manager is in a unique position to keep her finger on the pulse of the organization, and make sure that the organization is effective and efficient enough to make the best possible contribution to patients' health and to alleviating their suffering. A tall order!

19 Conclusion

As this book goes to press George Orwell's fictional year of 1984 has arrived; an opportune time, the reader may think, to be reminded that man-made systems and services should indeed be for the benefit of man. Health care, like any other social responsibility, has to remain within the domain of the human beings for whom it is designed.

Modern technology, with its more accurate means of recording information which in turn becomes more readily accessible, enables doctor and patient alike to benefit. Each may choose to shape the purposes of a comprehensive health-care service by placing future emphasis on education to prevent accidents and disease. The means to accomplish this are available; what is needed is the skilled and sensitive management of technical, financial, and human resources.

To regard health as a physical and psychological state where each individual can take an initiative may still seem a novel idea. Perhaps doctors and patients have preferred to collude with each other in creating too much dependency on experts with the awesome power of medicine. A well-managed, but nonetheless caring, health service must restore the balance so that patients and professionals are seen to share differing but complementary responsibilities. In his book *Limits to medicine*† Ivan Illich writes about the need for 'the recovery of personal responsibility for health care'. This will demand some changes in the aims and methods of a comprehensive service, where wider social and environmental factors will be seen to be linked to health.

Far from Orwell's 'Big Brother' world where people are slaves to the system, our contemporary information processing technology should help man to understand more about the nature of his environment and its relationship to his physical well being. More effective screening, more accurately collated personal histories, and better means to predict risks are well within the scope of a well-managed primary health care service.

In the past, there has been too much reliance on crisis management – waiting for things to go wrong. We hope that the preceding chapters have outlined some alternative pathways to planning the future we want. Different but complementary skills are needed. These skills include better ways of communicating and collaborating; better ways of diagnosing and solving problems; but perhaps most important of all – being prepared to look afresh at the way we do our work.

The prospect is exciting; the initiatives are ours; whether we are doctors, nurses, receptionists, social workers, patients – or managers.

† Illich, I. (1977) *Limits to medicine*, Penguin Books.

Appendices

Appendix A Procedure for immunization of infants and pre-school children

Schedule	Diphtheria/pertussis/tetanus injection	Poliomyelitis oral vaccine	Measles
1st	Age 3–4 months	3–4 months	12–15 months
2nd	Interval 8 weeks	Interval 8 weeks	–
3rd	Interval 4–6 months	Interval 4–6 months	–
Booster	(Diph./Tet.) 3–5 years	3–5 years	–

The immunization schedules may vary, but the one shown above is a current example. If no computer-based system is available, the following manual system can be used, in which the practice nurse or doctor does the injections, and claims are put in to the FPC for payment under the provisions of SFA ('Red Book') para. 27.

MASTER LIST OF CHILDREN UNDER ONE YEAR OF AGE

This list must be kept in an A4 book, by month of birth. The names can be obtained initially from the maternity records, and checked at the postnatal clinic. Any new arrivals to the practice under the age of one are similarly recorded, and those leaving deleted.

POSTNATAL VISIT

Mother is asked to sign the consent form for a complete course of injections. The child's card for application to go on the NHS list is completed (FP58); if not available, FP1 is completed. The mother is given an appointment for the first immunization. Immunization documents are completed for each child:

FP 74 – claim form;
FP111H – immunization record;
immunization record card for mother to keep;
consent form, which contains a list of contra-indications.

They are filed as described below. Those who do not attend are contacted by post, or health visitor's help is sought.

IMMUNIZATION FILE

A filing drawer with 13 suspended files is needed, marked for each month of the year, and 'overdue'. The 'overdue' file is at the front, then the current month's file, and so on in month order. If for example, the mother comes for a postnatal examination in February, and the first immunization is due in May, the documents are put in the file marked May, which is fifth file from the front.

First attendance

On attendance for the first immunization:
1. The child will be checked for fitness by doctor.
2. The mother will be questioned by the doctor or practice nurse as below:

Is the baby well today?
Has he or she ever had a fit or convulsion?
Has any close relative suffered with fits or convulsions?
Is baby having steroid or immuno-suppressive treatment?

These procedures are a medico-legal safeguard, and details may vary between districts. The advice of the District Community Physician may be sought.

If the answer to any of these questions is unsatisfactory, the doctor must decide before vaccine is given. Before measles vaccine, ask if child is allergic to egg.

3. Records are date stamped, batch numbers inserted, and then put in monthly file for next appointment, which is given to mother.

Later attendances

1. Similar procedures are adopted, with the additional question:

Was the child upset by the last injections?

2. If so, refer to doctor, and 'pertussis' element of vaccine will probably be omitted.

Each month

1. Scan last month's file for remaining records – put in 'overdue' file at front of drawer, and send appointment by post. If child is not brought for second appointment, mark in medical record and inform health visitor.

2. Put previous month's (empty) file at back.

3. When immunization course is complete, give mother the personal record card with approximate date for booster marked on it; file FP 111H in medical record, complete FP 74 and pass to doctor for signature, then send to FPC.

Appendix B Operational check-list for hypertension case finding

Operational check-list for hypertension case finding

1. Go through all practice notes.
2. Put red 'flag' in all those aged 20–70 (or agreed age limits).

Receptionist

1. When patient attends, check if blood pressure (BP) has been taken in past year.
2. If BP is less than 140/85 remove red flag and insert green flag, colour coded to represent 5 years hence. (If in doubt refer to practice nurse.)
3. Remainder – ask practice nurse to see patient to check BP before seeing doctor, if time allows and patient agrees.
4. New patients – insert red flag and refer to nurse.

Practice nurse

1. Take blood pressure in accordance with procedure in Hart (1980, Appendix 4, pp. 249–30).
2. If 'normal', remove red flag and insert green flag (colour code = 5 years hence).
3. If 'borderline' remove red flag and replace with appropriate colour for next year.
4. If 'raised', repeat twice at about weekly intervals. If subsequent reading is normal, proceed as above.
5. If still 'raised':
   (a) check urine for protein, glucose, and blood and record in notes;
   (b) take blood for blood count, urea, creatinine; and electrolytes;
   (c) do ECG, or have one done;
   (d) enquire about smoking habits and record in notes. Counsel appropriately and give handouts.
   (e) check weight and record in notes;
   (f) put blue sticker on outside of notes and remove red flag;
   (g) refer patient and record to doctor.

Doctor

1. Take history, including family history.
2. Check smoking habits and counsel.

3. Examine weight, heart, lungs, ankles, peripheral pulses, carotids, and fundi.

4. Check results of tests done by practice nurse and laboratory.

5. Discuss treatment plan with patient, and start it.

6. Arrange follow-up (not exceeding three monthly).

Follow-up

Fail-safe recall system needed so that defaulting does not escape notice.

1. *Receptionist* – to send appointment to see:

2. *Practice Nurse* who checks weight, BP, urine, and then see:

3. *Doctor* to re-check BP, adjust treatment, and make further follow-up appointment.

Review

1. *Clerk* – At end of first calendar year, get out all notes which still have a red flag. Pass them to:

2. *Practice Nurse*

(a) to check if normal BP has been recorded in past 5 years. If so, remove red flag and replace with appropriate colour for 5 years from date of reading.

(b) If no record, or BP raised or borderline, refer notes to doctor to decide on postal request to attend, *or nurse* to visit, *or doctor* to visit or telephone.

(c) Leave red flag in till patient attends.

Appendix C Planning a cervical cytology screening programme in a practice of 10 000 patients

THE INITIAL PLAN

1. Objective

To achieve maximum cervical cytology testing of the practice population in accordance with advice given by the Department of Health and Social Security (DHSS), with the aim of reducing mortality and morbidity from carcinoma of the cervix by early diagnosis and treatment.

2. Background information

Read Dr G. Lloyd's article in *Screening in general practice* pp. 317–27 (Hart 1975).

Cervical screening has DHSS support and it is recommended that it be carried out on all women 35 and over and on under 35s who have had three or more pregnancies. It is recommended that these tests should be repeated at five-year intervals or immediately following each quinquennial birthday, which ever comes first. For each test carried out as above, and for repeat tests at the request of the laboratory where the first smear was unsatisfactory, a fee of £8.20 (1988) will be paid on submitting form FP74 to the FPC (NHS General Medical Services, *Statement of fees and allowances* ('Red Book') para. 28–1 to 28–5, p. 36).

3. How can it be done?

Has anyone done this successfully? Enquire of local FPC if any practices are doing it systematically and visit them. Can their methods be applied here? Read references to successful programmes in general practice quoted above.

4. Method

Identify women at risk. This can be done from an age–sex register, if one exists, or by going through all the practice notes to select those over 35. Alternatively, a search of the FPC card-index of each doctor's patients might be quicker, if they agree. Women under 35 with three or more children could be identified from the notes, from health visitor records, or from maternity records. To identify those who have had three or more pregnancies would involve searching notes in order to include miscarriages and terminations of pregnancy, and this would take longer.

How long would each operation take? Do a pilot run on 100 notes. Could reception staff cope with extra load? Would the FPC co-operate? What is the likely cost of clerical work? It is likely that the number of women between 35 and 65 would be about 2000 in a practice of 10 000. If 100 per cent, consented this would involve about 33 tests per month.

Once a list of women at risk has been obtained, it is necessary to discover if they have had a cervical cytology test, and if so when. This involves going through their notes and marking the list with the date of the last test. Those who have had a hysterectomy or have persistently refused can be marked 'H' or 'R'.

Construct a recall diary, with one side of the page for each month. A ruled A4 size book of 144 pages would cover 10 years, which would suffice initially. Each page to be marked for month and year consecutively. Transfer names to the recall diary according to when next test is due (see para. 2). Include also the date of birth, address, and date of last test. How long will this take and at what cost?

5. Options

Construct the whole diary as a crash programme with extra help, or do it gradually with existing staff. Start with patients aged 35 and over and introduce the under-35s later, making a cut-off point at the age of 65. Alternatively, use a micro-computer.

6. Updating

Once the diary is complete, it would be advisable to introduce the names of those women between 30 and 35 who would become due in the next five-year period.

7. Sending for patients

Prepare an invitation with a patient's help, which can be duplicated and sent to those due for a test. If they do not respond mark case-notes 'cervical cytology test due' in red. Estimate the cost of postage. An alternative method is to mark in her notes the date the next test is due, so that she can be reminded if she turns up for some other reason.

8. Doing the tests

Tests can be done by a treatment-room sister with suitable training (see Jacka and Griffiths 1976), either in special sessions or by appointment in her ordinary sessions. She would complete Form FP74 which the patient and doctor would sign. Afterwards, she would be told when the next test was due (see para. 2) and an entry would be made in the cytology diary. The patient would be asked to call in or telephone for the result of the test.

An estimate can be made of the balance between fees earned and cost incurred, based on hypothetical 50 per cent or 75 per cent response rates.

Appendix D Geriatric survey: procedures

See sample proforma (p. 266).

Secretary

1. Prepare list of all patients over 70 or 75, for each doctor, from age/sex register or computer listing.

2. Pass list to doctor who will delete any who are already under supervision, or known refusals.

3. Fill in heading of proforma, attach to medical record, and pass to doctor at agreed rate (say four per week).

4. Record entry to geriatric survey on list.

Doctor

1. Complete Section A with relevant medical diagnoses problems.

2. Pass to health visitor for action.

Health visitor

1. Check medical record if necessary, e.g. hospital or social reports.
2. Return record for filing.
3. Complete social enquiry Section B, from own records.
4. If information missing, visit patient, and complete Section B.
5. Pass proforma to district nurse for action.

District nurse

1. Visit patient and explain purpose and nature of survey, request co-operation, and ensure that informed consent is given.

2. Enquire about symptoms using the following repertoire (Section C of proforma):

    (i) Is your appetite normal?
    (ii) Do you have indigestion or pain after meals?
        Do any foods upset your stomach?
    (iii) Is your weight steady now, or have you lost any weight recently?
    (iv) Do you have a cough? Do you cough up any sputum? Is it white, yellow or bloodstained?
    (v) Do you have any chest pain? Where is it situated? Is it made worse by exertion, or cold weather?

(vi) Are you short of breath when you exert yourself? (e.g. hurrying, climbing stairs).

(vii) Are any of your joints painful?

(viii) Do you have to get up at night to pass water? Is it ever painful? Do you have any difficulty in holding your water? (e.g. when you cough or sneeze). Have you ever had blood in the water?

(ix) Do you go to the toilet to pass a motion every day? Are you constipated? Is passing a motion painful? Do you ever have diarrhoea? Have you noticed blood in your motions? Have you ever passed black, tar-like motions?

(x) Have you had any bleeding from the back passage? (Females) Have you had discharge or bleeding from the front passage?

(xi) Have you any other symptoms or complaints? (Help patient to verbalize these.)

3. Please comment if patient has difficulty understanding the questions, or does not give reliable answers, or is mentally confused.

4. Put X in column if any *positive* symptoms and specify details.

5. Section D: Perform physical checks: †

(i) Test vision with card at three metres, with glasses. Specify if one or both eyes faulty.

(ii) Check mouth and specify if dental caries, or inadequate dentures, from the point of view of function.

(iii) Check hearing by quiet speech with each ear covered in turn. Check for wax with auriscope.

(iv) Check neck veins for rise of jugular venous pressure above clavicle.

(v) Check ankles for pitting oedema.

(vi) Check vibration sense in ankles; against tibial tuberosity and head of radius.

(vii) Examine feet for corns, callouses, and assess need for professional chiropody (instruct in home care of feet if relevant).

(viii) Obtain urine specimen at time of interview and check by uristix and culture at laboratory.
Arrange for later specimen to be collected using MSU technique (no Cetrimide).

(ix) Record blood pressure sitting. Take three readings and record.

(x) Check weight on portable scales.

(xi) Take blood for: haemoglobin, ESR, and urea and creatinine.
Record any other relevant observations.

---

† The district nurse will need the following equipment, and may need training in its use: vision testing card for use at 3 metres; pen torch; auriscope; tuning fork; blood pressure machine; stethoscope; portable scales; two bottles for urine sampling; Uristix or equivalent; 20 ml sterile syringe; needle; EDTA and fluoride bottles.

GERIATRIC SURVEY : PROFORMA

| Name | Surname | Forenames | M. S. W. |

Address: ....   GP ....

....   HV ....

D. of B ....

A. **Medical diagnoses/problems** (Dr to list)   *Date of diagnoses*
   1.
   2.
   3.
   4.
   5.
   6.

B. **1st visit   Health Visitor †**   Date ....

   Accommodation: House/flat/bungalow/caravan/other
   Facilities:
   Social contacts/isolation:
   Does impaired mental state affect independence?   YES/NO
   Does poor motivation affect independence?   YES/NO
   Does impairment of vision, speech, or hearing   YES/NO
   affect independence

   Is patient INDEPENDENT for: Comments
   Mobility indoors   YES/NO
   Mobility outdoors   YES/NO
   Dressing   YES/NO
   Food   YES/NO
   Toilet   YES/NO
   Bathing   YES/NO
   Household tasks   YES/NO
   Finance   YES/NO
   Aids
   Treatments

C. **2nd visit   District Nurse**   Date
   Symptomatic enquiry   (Mark X if present)
   1. Poor appetite
   2. Indigestion
   3. Loss of weight
   4. Productive cough
   5. Substernal pain
   6. Short of breath
   7. Painful joints
   8. Abnormal micturition
   9. Difficulty with bowels or diarrhoea
   10. Rectal or vaginal bleeding
   11. Other symptoms – please list

   ....

   ....

D. **Physical checks**

   1. Visual acuity (with glasses)– worse than 6/60
                                      worse than 6/18
                                      6/18 or better

   2. Dental problem
   3. Hearing loss (check with auriscope)
   4. Jugular venous pressure raised
   5. Oedema of ankles
   6. Vibration sense lost in feet
   7. Needs chiropody (examine feet)
   8. Urine – contains protein
                 contains glucose
                 MSU sent to lab.
   9. Blood pressure (sitting) (Systolic)
       Repeat if raised   (Diastolic (phase 5)

  10. Weight
  11. Blood taken for FBC
                     ESR
                     Urea/creatinine

Other observations:

....

....

E. **List of current medication** (include self-medication)

Name of drug or medicine	Size or quantity	No, of times daily

F. **3rd visit**   **Doctor**

Date ....

Examine heart   normal/abnormal   ....
Examine lungs   normal/abnormal   ....
Examine abdomen   normal/abnormal   ....

Other systems indicated by questionnaire:

....

....

Daily quantity smoked ? ....
Daily alcohol consumption ? ....

Doctor update problem list A.
Action recommended: By whom ?

....

....

....

Review interval: .... months
                 .... years

† It is important that the health visitors' social enquiry form corresponds with the one she normally uses. These questions are taken from the form used by Oxfordshire District Health Authority (Teaching).

6. Section E: List all tablets, capsules, or medicine taken by patient, including self-medication. Complete column of number per day from patient's answer.

7. When form complete, pass to secretary.

Secretary

1. Collect laboratory results and clip to proforma. Attach to medical record and pass to doctor for action.

2. Arrange surgery appointment if mobile. Put on visiting list if not mobile.

Doctor

1. Check survey and laboratory results.
2. Visit patient.
3. Examine heart, lungs, abdomen, and other systems if indicated.
4. Ask and record tobacco and alcohol intake.
5. Update problem list A.
6. Record action recommended and by whom.
7. Record review interval.
8. Discuss with health visitor or district nurse if needed.
9. Pass to secretary.

Secretary

1. Pass messages about action.
2. Diary when action completed, or remind.
3. Diary review interval.
4. File proforma in medical record.

Appendix E Books written for patients

'THE FACTS' SERIES, OXFORD UNIVERSITY PRESS

Ageing
Nicholas Coni, William Davison,
and Stephen Webster
AIDS
A. J. Pinching
Alcoholism
Donald W. Goodwin
Arthritis and rheumatism
J. T. Scott
Asthma
(second edition)
Donald Lane and Anthony Storr
Back pain
Malcolm Jayson
Blindness and visual handicap
John H. Dobree and Eric Boulter
Blood disorders
Sheila T. Callender
Breast cancer
Michael Baum
Cancer
Sir Ronald Bodley Scott
Childhood diabetes
J. O. Craig
Contraception
P. Bromwich and A. D. Parsons
Coronary heart disease
J. P. Shillingford
Cystic fibrosis
A. Harris and M. Super
Eating disorders
(second edition) S. Abraham and
D. Llewellyn-Jones

Epilepsy
Anthony Hopkins
Hip replacement
Kevin Hardinge
Hypothermia
K. J. Collins
Kidney disease
Stewart Cameron
Liver disease and gallstones
A. G. Johnson and D. Triger
Lung cancer
C. J. Williams
Migraine
F. Clifford Rose and M. Gawel
Miscarriage
G. C. L. Lachelin
Multiple sclerosis
(second edition) Bryan Matthews
Parkinson's disease
Gerald Stern and Andrew Lees
Phobia
Donald W. Goodwin
Rabies
(second edition) Edited by C. Kaplan
Schizophrenia
Ming Tsuang
Sexually transmitted diseases
David Barlow
Stroke
F. Clifford Rose and R. Capildeo
Thyroid disease
R. I. S. Bayliss

PENGUIN BOOKS

Titles include:
Alcoholism
Anorexia nervosa
Baby and child
Babyhood
Care of the dying
The emergency book

N. Kessel and H. Walton
R. L. Palmer
Penelope Leach
Penelope Leach
Richard Lamerton
B. Smith and G. Stevens

The experience of breast feeding	Sheila Kitzinger
The experience of childbirth	Sheila Kitzinger
From woman to woman	Lucienne Lanson
Boys and sex	Wardell Pomeroy
Girls and sex	Wardell Pomeroy
How to lose weight	Michael Spira
Medicines. A guide for everybody	Peter Parish (4th Edn.)
Our bodies ourselves	Boston Womens Health Collective
Ourselves and our children	Boston Womens Health Collective
A patient's guide to operations	David Delvin
Physical fitness	Royal Canadian Airforce
Treat yourself to sex	Paul Brown and Carolyn Faulder
Work and health	Andrew Melhuish

PAN BOOKS

Understanding cystitis	Angela Kilmartin
You and your back	David Delvin
Life change—the menopause	Barbara Evans
Not all in the mind (allergy)	Richard Mackarness
Taking the rough with the smooth	Andrew Stanway

FAMILY DOCTOR PUBLICATIONS (37 titles)

List available from BMA House, Tavistock Square, London WC1H 9JP.

HEALTH EDUCATION AUTHORITY (England, Wales, and Northern Ireland)

Publishes many excellent pamphlets and posters, including some in Asian and Welsh languages, and Health Education News. List may be obtained from Hamilton House, Mabledon Place, London WC1H 9TX, or from the health education unit of the local Health Authority. Most of the publications are issued free. Tel. 01 631 0930.

SCOTTISH HEALTH EDUCATION GROUP

Woodburn House, Canaan's Lane, Edinburgh, EH10 4SG. Tel. 031-447-8044.

WOMEN'S HEALTH CONCERN

Seymour Street, London, W1H 5WB. Titles include:
Sexually transmitted diseases
The menopause
Post-natal depression
Pre-menstrual syndrome and period pains

GEORGE ALLEN & UNWIN

Take care of yourself, by J. A. Muir Gray and S. Small
A practical do-it-yourself guide to medical care.

POSITIVE HEALTH GUIDE, Martin Dunitz, London.

Stress and relaxation, by Jane Madders.
Don't forget fibre in your diet, by Denis Burkitt.
Other books available on back pain, arthritis, heart disease, and asthma.

Appendix F Useful addresses

The Association of Health Centre and Practice Administrators (AHCPA)
  Lord Lister Health Centre,
  121 Wood Grange Road,
  London E7 0EP.
  Tel. 01-555 5331

The Association of Medical Secretaries, Practice Administrators and Receptionists (AMSPAR)
  Tavistock House South,
  Tavistock Square,
  London WC1H 9LN.
  Tel. 01-387 6005

British Medical Association
  BMA House,
  Tavistock Square,
  London WC1H 9JB.
  Tel. 01-387 4499

BMA Regional Offices
  Scotland: Tel. 041-332 1862
  Wales: Tel. 0222-485336
  N. Ireland: Tel. 0232-649 065

Bureau of Medical Practitioner Affairs Ltd.
  Rigby Hall,
  Rigby Lane,
  Bromsgrove B60 2EW.
  0527–78370 (or 01-699 6688)

Department of Health and Social Security (General Practice Division)
  Eileen House,
  80–94 Newington Causeway,
  London SE1 6BY.
  Tel. 01-703 6380

General Practice Finance Corporation
  Tavistock House North,
  Tavistock Square,
  London WC1 9JL.
  Tel. 01-387 5274

Health Services Management Centre
  The University of Birmingham,
  Park House,
  40 Edgbaston Park Road,
  Birmingham B15 2RT.
  Tel. 021-455 7511

Information Resources Centre (RCGP)
  14 Princes Gate,
  London SW7 1PU.
  Tel. 01-581 3232

Institute of Health Service Managers
  75 Portland Place,
  London W1N 4AN.
  Tel. 01-580 5041

King's Fund Centre Library
  (Librarian: Ms Sue Cook)
  126 Albert Street,
  London NW1 7NF.
  Tel. 01-267 6111

King's Fund College
  (Librarian: Nancy Black)
  2 Palace Court,
  London W2 4HS.
  Tel. 01-727 0581

Royal College of General Practitioners
  14 Princes Gate,
  London SW7 1PU.
  Tel. 01-581 3232

Royal College of Nurses (UK)
  Henrietta Place,
  London W1M 0AB.
  Tel. 01-580 2646

Scottish Home and Health Department
  New St. Andrew's House,
  St. James' Centre,
  Edinburgh EH1 3TB.
  Tel. 031-556 8400

FILMS, VIDEOTAPE AND TAPE-SLIDE PROGRAMMES

Graves Medical Audiovisual Library
  Holly House,
  220 New London Road,
  Chelmsford,
  Essex CM2 9BJ.
  Tel. 0245 83351

M.S.D. Foundation
  Tavistock House,
  Tavistock Square,
  London WC1H 9JZ.
  Tel. 01-387 6881

Video-Arts Ltd.
  Dumbarton House,
  68 Oxford Street,
  London W1N 9LA.
  Tel. 01-637 7288

British Life Assurance Trust for Health Education (BLITHE)
  BLAT Centre,
  BMA House,
  Tavistock Square,
  London WC1H 9JP.

See also p. 82

DATA PROTECTION

Data Protection Registrar
  Springfield House,
  Water Lane,
  Wilmslow,
  Cheshire SK9 5AX.

Information also obtainable from Information Resources Centre and British Medical Association, see p. 271.

Appendix G Further reading list on management

Allen, D. and Grimes, D. (1982). *Management for clinicians.* Pitman, London.
A guide on the role which doctors can play in the management of the National Health Service. Mainly refers to consultants, but one chapter for GPs.

Drury, M. (1986). *Medical secretary's and receptionist's Handbook* (5th Edn.). Baillière, London.
The standard text book for practice secretaries. Strongly recommended.

Eskin, F. (1981). *Doctors and management skills.* MCB Publications, Bradford.
A useful management primer for doctors in NHS management.

Handy, C. (1978). *Gods of management. Who they are, how they work and why they will fail.* Pan Books, London.
A tongue-in-cheek look at the conflict between individual and organizational needs.

Jones, R. V. H. *et al.* (1985). *Running a practice,* 3rd Edn. An expanded text of the course for GPs at Exeter. Croom Helm, London. A valuable guide.

Open Systems Group (1981). *Systems behaviour,* 3rd Edn. (Formerly Beishon, J. and Peters, G.). Published for the Open University by Harper & Row, London.
A clear and comprehensive guide to the concept of systems.

Pritchard, P. M. M. (1981). *Manual of primary health care. Its nature and organization,* 2nd Edn. Oxford University Press.
Written primarily for GP trainees. A companion volume to this book.

Sidney, E., Brown, M., and Argyle, M. (1973). *Skills with people. A guide for managers.* Hutchinson, London. A readable text to supplement the first five chapters of this book. Strongly recommended.

Stewart, R. (1979). *The reality of management.* Pan Books, London.
An up-to-date and readable account of the application of management theory.

The Industrial Society. *Notes for managers.*
A comprehensive Series of booklets for managers, costing about £1.50 each. They are strongly recommended. Examples of titles are listed below:
   Decision taking.
   Delegation.
   Effective use of time.
   Guide to employment practices.
   The manager's responsibility for communication.
   The manager's guide to target setting.
   Selection interviewing.
   Guide to effective meetings.
   Guide to using the telephone.
   Motivation.
Available from: The Industrial Society, Publications Department, Freepost, London, SW1Y 5BR.

The British Institute of Management publishes a series of Management Checklists covering similar topics to those listed above. They are brief, but have a list of books for further reading. Available from: Publication Sales, The British Institute of Management, Management House, Parker Street, London, WC2B 5PT.

References

Alarcon, R. de (1969). A personal medical reference index. *Lancet,* **i**, 301–5.

Anderson, P. *et al.* (1980). A broader training for medical receptionists. *J. R. Coll. Gen. Pract.* **26**, 379; **30**, 490–4.

Anderson, W. and Steel, R. (1979). The general practitioner and the receptionist. *Practitioner* **223**, 603–8.

Arber, S. and Sawyer, L. (1982). Do appointment systems work. *Br. med. J.* **284**, 478–80.

Balint, M. *et al.* (1970). *Treatment or diagnosis. A study of repeat prescriptions in general practice.* Tavistock Publications, London.

Beishon, J. and Peters, G. (1981). *Systems behaviour,* 3rd Edn. See Open Systems Group.

Bull, M. J. V. (1982). Practising prevention. Contraception. *Br. med. J.* **284**, 1535.

Byrne, P. and Long, B. E. (1976). *Doctors talking to patients. A study of the verbal behaviour of general practitioners consulting in their surgeries.* HMSO, London.

Cartwright, A. and Anderson, R. (1981). *General practice revisited. A second study of patients and their doctors.* Tavistock Publications, London.

Cullinan, A. and Ellis, N. (1982). Health and safety at Work Act 1974. (three articles). *Br. med. J.* **285**, 1323, 1379, 1467.

DHSS (1981*a*). *The primary health care team.* Report of a joint working group of the standing medical, nursing and midwifery advisory committees. (Harding–Frost report). HMSO, London.

—— (1981*b*). *Handbook for receptionists.* P.O. Box 21, Stanmore, Middlesex, HA7 1AY: £3.70.

Doll, R. and Peto, R. (1981). *The causes of cancer.* Oxford University Press.

Drucker, P. (1974). *Management.* Heinemann, London.

Drury, M. (1986). *The medical secretary and receptionist's handbook,* 5th Edn. Baillière Tindall, London.

Ellis, N. (1987). *Employing staff,* 2nd Edn. British Medical Association, London.

Fowler, G. and Gray, J. A. M. (1982). *Prevention in general practice.* Oxford University Press.

Fuller, J. H. S. and Toon, P. D. (1988). *Medical practice in a multicultural society.* Heinemann Medical, Oxford.

Gilmore, M., Bruce, N., and Hunt, M. (1974). *The work of the nursing team in general practice.* Central Council for the Education and Training of Health Visitors, London.

Hannay, D. R. (1979). *The symptom iceberg. A study of community health.* Routledge & Kegan Paul, London.

Harris, T. A. (1973). *I'm O.K.–you're O.K.* Pan Books, London.

Hart, C. R. (ed.) (1975). *Screening in general practice.* Churchill Livingstone, Edinburgh.

Hart, J. T. (1980). *Hypertension.* Churchill Livingstone, Edinburgh.

—— (1981). A new kind of doctor. *J. R. Soc. Med.* **74**, 871–83.

Henley, A. (1979). *Asian patients in hospital and at home.* King Edwards Hospital Fund for London/Pitman Medical.

Huntington, J. (1981). *Social work and general medical practice: collaboration or conflict.* John Allen and Unwin, London.

Jacka, S. M. and Griffiths, D. G. (1976). *Treatment room nursing. A handbook for nursing sisters working in general practice.* Blackwell Scientific Publications, Oxford.

Jones, R. V. H. *et al.* (1985). *Running a practice,* 3rd Edn. Croom Helm, London.

Kaprio, L. (1979). *Primary health care in Europe.* Euro reports and studies No. 14. World Health Organization, Regional Office for Europe, Copenhagen.

Kepner, C. H. and Tregoe, B. B. (1981). *The new rational manager.* Princeton Research Press, New Jersey.

King, J. (1983). Health beliefs in the consultation. *Essays on doctor–patient communication* (eds. D. Pendleton and J. Hasler). Academic Press, London.

Likert, R. (1967). *The human organization.* McGraw-Hill, New York.

Lucas, S. B. and Metcalfe, D. (1982). *Computers in general practice. Computer working party interim advice.* Royal College of General Practitioners, London.

Mapes, R. (1980). *Prescribing practice and drug usage.* Croom Helm, London.

Marsh, G. N. (1981). Stringent prescribing in general practice. *Br. med. J.* **283**, 1159–60.

Marson, W. S. *et al.* (1973). Measuring the quality of general practice. *J. R. Coll. Gen. Pract.* **23**, 23.

Metcalfe, D. (1982). Information systems and general practice. *Computers and the general practitioner* (eds. A. Malcolm and J. Poyser). Pergamon Press, Oxford.

NCC (1982). *Patients' rights. A guide to the rights and responsibilities of patients and doctors in the NHS.* National Consumer Council, 18 Queen Anne's Gate. London, S.W.1. Obtainable (£1.50) from local community health council. [Republished HMSO (1983).]

OHE (1980). *Medicines. 50 years of progress.* Office of Health Economics, London.

Open systems Group (1981). *Systems behaviour,* 3rd edn. Published for Open University by Harper and Row, London. (Previously published under Beishon and Peters.)

Pendleton, D. (1981). Patients' views of general practice. Quoted in editorial *J. R. Coll. Gen. Pract.* **246**, 5–7 (1983).

Pike, L. A. (1980). Teaching parents about child health using a practice booklet. *J. R. Coll. Gen. Pract.* **30**, 517–19.

—— (1981). A by-pass card for infants. *Practitioner* **225**, 956–7.

—— (1982). Organizing health education. *Br. med. J.* **284**, 874–5.

Pritchard, P. M. M. (1981). *Manual of primary health care,* 2nd edn. Oxford University press.

—— (1983). Patient participation. In *Medical annual* (ed. D. P. Gray). Wright, Bristol.

RCGP (1964). Report on colour tagging by research committee of council. *J. R. Coll. Gen. Pract.* **viii**, 94–5.

—— (1972). *The future general practitioner. Learning and teaching.* Royal College of General Practitioners and British Medical Journal, London.

—— (1981*a*). *Patient participation in general practice. A collection of essays.* (ed. P. M. M. Pritchard). Royal College of General Practitioners, London. £3.45.

—— (1981*b*). *Health and prevention in primary care.* Report from General Practice, No. 18. London.

—— (1981*c*). *Prevention of arterial disease.* Report from General Practice, No. 19, London.

—— (1981*d*). *Prevention of psychiatric disorders in general practice.* Report from General Practice, No. 20. London.

—— (1981*e*). *Family planning. An exercise in preventive medicine.* Report from General Practice, No. 21. London.

Rubin, I. Plovnick, M., and Fry, R. (1975). *Improving the co-ordination of care. A program for health team development.* Ballinger, Cambridge, MA.

Russell, M. A. H. *et al.* (1979). Effect of general practitioner's advice against smoking. *Br. med. J.* **2**, 231–5.

Stewart, R. (1979). *The reality of management/organizations.* Pan Books, London.

Tannenbaum, R. and Schmidt, W. H. (1958). How to choose a leadership pattern. *Harv. Bus. Rev.* **36**(2), 95–101.

Tulloch, A. J. (1981). Repeat prescribing for elderly patients. *Br. med. J.* **282**, 1647–54.

Vaill, P. B. (1982). The purposing of high-performing systems. *Organizational dynamics.* Autumn 1982. AMACOM periodicals division, American Management Associations.

Whyte, W. H. (1956). *The organization man.* Simons & Schuster.

Winthrop Laboratories (1982). *General Practitioner Year Book.*

WHO/UNICEF (1978). *Primary health care.* Report of the International Conference on Primary Health Care, Alma-Ata 1978. World Health Organization, Geneva.

WHO (1981). *Managerial process for national health development.* Health for all series, No. 5. World Health Organization, Geneva.

Wilcock, G., Gray, J. A. M. and Pritchard, P. M. M. (1982). *Geriatric problems in general practice.* Oxford University Press.

Williamson, J. D. and Danahar, K. (1977). *Self care in health.* Croom Helm, London.

Zander, L. I., Beresford, S. A. A., and Thomas, P. (1978). *Medical records in general practice.* Occasional Paper No. 5. Royal College of General Practitioners, London.

Index